The Great Little Book of Yoga Stories

Yoga Philosophy for All Ages

Book 1

TESSA HILLMAN

First published online in 2008 by www.yogastories.co.uk

Second Edition Published by SifiPublishing, 2019

Third Edition Published by Top of the Village Publishing, 2022

Re-print 2022 Publisher Top of the Village Publishing

topofthevillagepublishing.co.uk

Contact: tessa.hillman2@gmail.com

Website: yogastories.co.uk

This book is a simplified and updated version of *Guptananda's Stories, Yoga Philosophy for Young people* pub 2008.

ISBN: Paperback 978-1-910088-66-1

ISBN: ebook 978-1-910088-67-8

Illustration: Alan Nisbet, Tessa Hillman
and Sally Atkins www.sallyatkinsartist.co.uk

Cover design: Mick Clough handmade-media.co.uk

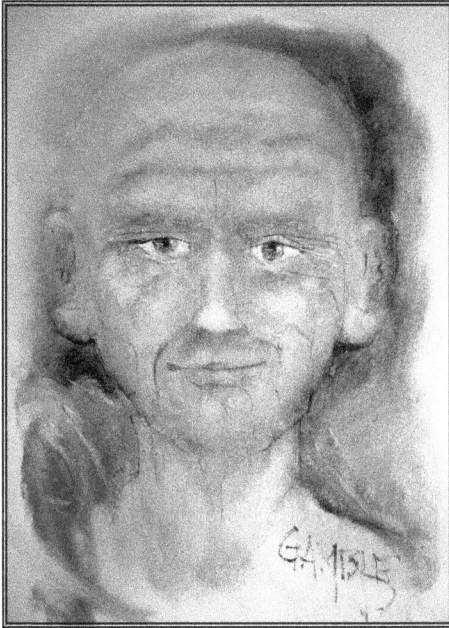

Swami Ramesh Guptananda

Portrait by Patrick Gamble, psychic artist

painted April 2002

CONTENTS

INTRODUCTION

Here is a book all young yoga fans need to read. It is a new look at old wisdom; an easy first step on the road to 'enlightenment', or understanding what life is really about. It's handy for yoga teachers too – ideal for the first forays into yoga philosophy for your classes.

The ancient scriptures are wonderful, but there are a lot of words and meanings that can be very difficult to grasp. Here, though, are simple short stories to make you smile, think and learn. They are told in the voice of an Indian guru, *Swami** Ramesh Guptananda. Imagine you can hear his voice as you read them. They show, through talking about his life, what the 'rules of life' are and how to follow them.

The original 'rules' came from the sage*, Patanjali, many hundreds of years ago. They still apply to this day.

I have included a 'New words' list (those with a star* in the text) at the end of each story to encourage you to read the stories and to increase your vocabulary* at the same time.

The questions at the end of each story will help you to think about how the stories remind you of aspects of your own life and help you to learn from *Swami** Guptananda's tales. You don't need to be religious to enjoy this book; it is not about religion, it is about living well.

NEW WORDS:

Swami: teacher

Sage: very wise person

Vocabulary: a list of words and their meanings

These stories are brought to you by a yoga teacher who likes to meditate and to ask for help with her teaching. Fair enough. Many of us do this do we not? We send up a prayer or a thought that we hope perhaps someone in the 'beyond' might hear. What came to this teacher came in the voice of Guptananda. The stories are all about him. Sometimes he talks as if he is telling the story about another person – it is as if he is slightly ashamed or embarrassed to admit that he did such things. After all, should not a *guru* be perfect? But he always admits the truth. We always know that the tale was about him. So don't let him confuse you. Just go with it.

Guptananda was only human and had to learn from his mistakes, like all of us do. Don't be afraid to make mistakes, you will certainly learn from them, or at least you will go on repeating the same mistake until you do learn from it!

Enjoy the stories!

All *Sanskrit* words are in italics for clarity.

NOTES FOR YOGA TEACHERS

There are several ways to use this book.

1. Read the book yourself and meditate upon those subjects which jump out at you. Do they reflect areas that could do with some attention in your life?

2. Read some of the shorter stories to your students or your children.

3. Choose one of the laws at a time, and work with it for a week or a month, on yourself, in your classes, or with your family.

4. Precis some of the longer stories, putting them into your own words, not giving the whole game away. You may give your students an

appetite to read the book and benefit from it for themselves.

Different stories will become relevant at different ages as children mature through their teens. This is a good book to go back to year after year.

Book Two will consist of stories on the Eight Limbs of Yoga, the *Gunas* and the *Chakras*. It will be published some months after Book One and will be especially useful to new or aspiring yoga teachers.

The *Swami* Guptananda said: 'There is no point in teaching your students spiritual practices unless they are following the rules of life, or the *Yamas* and *Niyamas*.' This can be difficult when your students are more mature and often many years older than you, the teacher. This is where stories come in so handy – you are not preaching, you are giving food for thought, and perhaps offering students material that may be useful for their own children or grandchildren.

ABOUT
GUPTANANDA

Guptananda always enjoyed helping others. Even as a small child he was deeply affected by other people's needs. He had a gentle sense of humour and kindness about him that draws us into his stories. He didn't mind laughing at his own mistakes. This book is full of stories about his life from the age of four until his mid-twenties.

Ramesh Guptananda and his family lived very many years ago in Northern India in a comfortable house with grounds and servants' quarters. They were *Brahmins* (from the priestly class) and his father was the chief scribe at the temple. His mother organised the servants at home. Five servants looked after the house and grounds. Ramesh had a brother called Anil who was born two years after him and a sister Usha who was four years younger than Ramesh. His family called him Ramu until he became 'too important' for pet names!

Ramesh was very proud to have a horse, Raja, whom he loved dearly and who features in some of the stories.

At the age of sixteen, Ramesh decided to follow a spiritual path. He found a guru who was willing to take him on, who he lived and travelled with, but in his twenties he thought that family life would suit him better. His uncle arranged a family gathering where he met a lovely girl, Meera, and they were married within a few short months. Ramesh then worked alongside his father as a scribe in the temple. After ten years of a very happy marriage, sadly, Meera died, and we know no more about his life from then on, except that he returned to the path of the holy man living with his own guru, travelling and advising people on their spiritual growth.

These tales are centred around family, temple and village life, providing funny or touching incidents which show us how the 'values' or 'rules of life' apply to everyday living.

THE *YAMAS* AND *NIYAMAS* – THE RULES OF LIFE

These are rules about things we should not do and things we should do.

The *Yamas*, or the Restraints, are the things we should not do.

The *Niyamas*, or the Observances, are the things we should do.

CHAPTER 1

THE *YAMAS*

The *Yamas*, or the Restraints: the things we should not do:

Yama 1: Non-violence – *Ahimsa* – We should not be violent.

Yama 2: Truth – *Satya* – We should not tell lies.

Yama 3: Non-stealing – *Asteya* – We should not steal.

Yama 4: Chastity – *Bramacharya* – We should keep our sexuality under control.

Yama 5: Non-greed – *Aparigraha* – We should not be greedy.

There are more rules, but these are considered to be the main ones. We will look at some others in Chapter 3.

STORY 1

Yama 1: Non-violence – Ahimsa

WHO CAN JUMP THE HIGHEST?

The young man who features in most of these stories had quite a colourful life. As a scholar, he always enjoyed competing with others in feats of courage and daring, as well as in his academic* studies. One day, he and his friends were seeing who could jump the highest. One friend became very angry, because everyone else had beaten him and he liked to think that he was the best. He began to lash out and hit our young man saying that he had cheated and that he wanted to fight him to prove that he was indeed the best, the strongest and, yes, that he could jump the highest too! Our young man was very surprised at this outburst*, but agreed to meet the other after the studies were over later in the day. Just as the two youngsters had begun their scrap the teacher appeared.

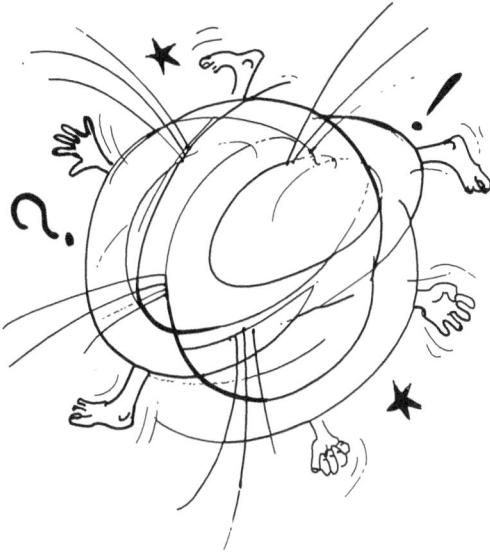

"What is this?" he said. "Do I see you, Ramesh Guptananda, fighting again? What is it about this time?"

The boys stopped shamefacedly[*] and explained the argument to the teacher. The wise old man laughed and said: "People try to prove all sorts of things with violence. They try to prove that they are more gifted, stronger, or cleverer. They try to prove that they have more rights to land, or possessions, or women, but I have never heard of fighting to prove that someone can jump higher than another person! Now, boys, there is always a better way to show the truth than to resort to fisticuffs*. Violence is never the answer. It diminishes* the perpetrator* rather than proving him the deserving victor*. Please do not resort to it again! I would like you to come to my room together tomorrow morning to tell me how you are going to resolve this argument in a civilised manner."

$\oplus$

NEW WORDS

Academic: having to do with school or what you learn in school

Diminishes: makes smaller

Fisticuffs: fighting with fists

Outburst: a sudden explosion of strong feeling, such as anger

Perpetrator: a person who does something wrong

Shamefacedly: expressing shame, embarrassed

Victor: winner

Some questions to ask yourself:

? How may violence affect the victim?

? How might a violent person feel about themself?

? How would it be if everyone used violence to solve problems?

? What sort of world would we have if everyone was non-violent?

Yama 2: Truth – *Satya*

THE PRINCE WHO
DID NOT SPEAK

When I was first married, I wanted to impress my young wife with my wisdom and other qualities. She was very much in love with me, as indeed I was with her. I used to work as a scribe in the temple and though not a priest, I had a certain amount of respect paid to me by many of the worshippers. One day, I thought I would tell my wife how they treated me, but I got carried away. I told her that the local prince had visited with a number of his dignitaries* (as he had, but on a day when I was actually running an errand in another part of the town). I told her that he had offered me '*namaste*'*, a respectful gesture, and that he had spoken to me.

24

"What did he say?" she asked eagerly. But it was too late. My guilt had overcome me. I blushed and stammered and told her I could not remember. I turned away, worried by my dishonesty, but still determined to show her how important I felt I had become. She looked at me quizzically*.

"Ah, yes," I continued, "the prince told me that ours was a very beautiful temple and that the writings were very well presented." I felt myself blush to the very roots of my hair. I glanced back at my wife half-hoping she hadn't heard me, or noticed my blushes.

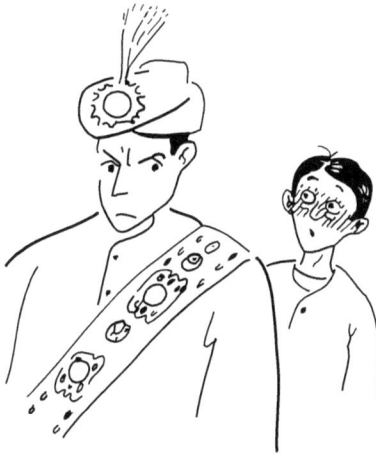

She looked at me long and hard, then she said, "I know you were not at temple the day before yesterday, because you told me what you had to do before you set off for work. I, on the other hand, was at temple and I watched the prince throughout the course of his visit. Neither were you there, nor did the prince offer 'namaste'* to any of the priests, staff or worshippers. Shame on you, my husband! Do you not think that I love you enough? Do you really think that you need to impress me to make me love you more? Well I do not love you less for having lied to me, but please do not do it again!"

NEW WORDS

Dignitaries: those who hold a high office or rank

Namaste: a greeting of respect made to another person; the hands are held in the prayer position in front of the chest

Quizzically: puzzled, expressing doubt, confusion or questioning

Some questions to ask yourself:

? How important is it that you can trust your friends and family to be honest and speak the truth?

? How do you feel about yourself when you tell lies?

? Why do people tell lies? Can you think of some different kinds of lies that people tell?

? Are all lies equally bad?

? Sometimes people tell lies when they are afraid, or when they are feeling 'not good enough'. Can you think of some examples of this and of how to solve the problem in a more honest way?

If we can be trusted to speak the truth and can trust others to do the same then we all know where we stand.

STORY 3

Yama 2: Truth – *Satya*

THE PEBBLE

In the old days, when my father seemed like a god to me and I was perhaps seven years of age, a young man came to stay with us. He was a distant relative and Father had told his parents that he would be welcome to live with us for a while, to discover whether he liked the work in the temple. He would go in with Father every day and be introduced to all the other temple workers. Father would instruct him in calligraphy – the careful writing of the scriptures* – and would explain the meaning of the verses to him. He would be with us for six months.

Now I had two 'gods' in my household. This young man was so clever, it seemed to me; so beautiful and so funny. I followed him everywhere hoping to learn a trick or two perhaps. When he smiled I felt that I would melt. His face became radiant like the sun. Everyone loved him. Father had great hopes for him. Not only could he write beautifully, he could also draw. When he had finished his writing he would often draw a beautiful design at the bottom of his work. On his days off he would take pen and paper and sit in some corner of our grounds and draw the flowers and the trees; sometimes he drew us, the children in my family. He gave me a beautiful picture of my sister and myself sitting by the well. How I treasured it. I asked one of the workmen to make a frame for it and I displayed it in our house for all to behold*.

Late one evening, a messenger came to call the young man away. His father had died and he had to return home to look after his family. We were all distraught*. Our lovely visitor was leaving. How we would miss him! My little sister didn't really understand that he would be leaving for ever. Maybe nobody told her, but they told me. I wanted to cry. Perhaps I did cry? There would be a large gap in my life. Who would teach me all the games and jokes now? Father was too busy, Mother didn't know many games or jokes and the servants' jokes never seemed very funny to me.

Father had told us that our friend would be leaving early the following morning. I ran away to hide my sorrow and wondered what I could do to show him how I loved him and to make him come back. I couldn't think of anything at all. I couldn't think of the words or any present that I could give him. Then I remembered a story he had told us. It was about a stone in the stream that ran past our stables. It was a lovely smooth stone and he told us that when it started life it had been rough and ugly. Through its life it had learnt many things and its rough edges had been worn away by all the other stones it had met. Gradually it became more beautiful. The smoother it became the more its lovely colours shone through and when it lay at the bottom of the stream with the sun shining on it, it glowed like a jewel.

I picked up a very smooth stone out of the stream; it had amber and red stripes running through it. It was very pretty. I decided to give it to our friend. I wanted to tell him the truth about what I felt for him, but I couldn't find the words. The stone would have to do it for me.

I shyly gave the stone to him before he left. His eyes lit up. Thinking of his story he said, "I shall keep this to remember you by, Ramu. To me you are already like this pretty stone. Many

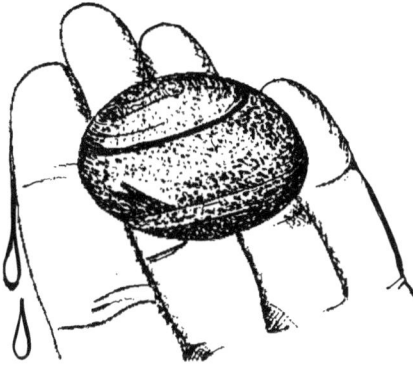

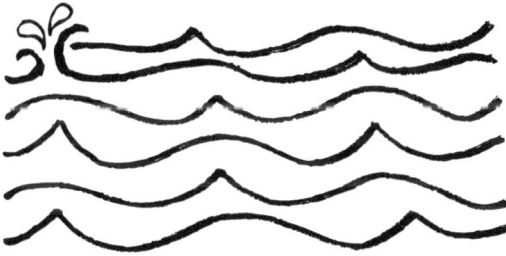

lifetimes have already rubbed the rough edges off you, but there is still much to learn. Unlike this little stone you will grow bigger. It would be dishonest of me to say that you will have no rough edges to be rubbed off. Every boy of seven has a whole lifetime of experience ahead to polish him up, but I think you will not find the polishing process too painful as you are quite well rounded already."

I did not really understand the truth behind

my friend's words, but I always remembered them. Now, looking back, I see that my struggles were not as difficult as those of many I encountered* and for that I was grateful.

When troubles came to me I would think of that stone and think of the troubles as another step in the process of being polished up to a beautiful finish!

$\oplus$

You may be asking what the Pebble Story has to do with truth. There are several truths in it. One is that young Ramesh could not find words to say how he felt about his friend, so he gave the pebble to show the truth.

Another is about what people believe. Some believe that we are here on Earth for a purpose and that is to learn certain things and to take the knowledge of those things with us into our next life when we return in a different body.

Others believe we only have one life on Earth and after that we may go to Heaven. Still others believe that when we die there is nothing left behind except the memories that other people have of us.

Whichever of those may be true, it is certain that we learn from our mistakes, if we are wise, and our 'rough edges' are rubbed off in the process!

The truth is that we must respect other people's beliefs, because it is impossible to prove what really happens after death and, who knows, there might be several different answers.

Yama 3: Non-stealing – Asteya

RAJA IS STOLEN

A very long time ago, before cars were invented and men travelled on foot, or by mule or horse, or even carried each other, there was a young man. Could it have been me, Guptananda?

This young man had a lovely black horse called Raja. It was not perfectly black, having a white patch, which hardly showed, under one fetlock*. The young man greatly treasured his horse, which he kept in a stable next door to his house. One day, very early, before dawn, he heard the sound of muffled horse's hooves on the cobbled steps outside his house. He tiptoed outside to discover a thief who had wrapped the horse's feet in leathers and was leading it away into the darkness. Our young man was so furious that he leapt out of the shadows, straight onto Raja's back. The horse, recognizing his master's voice, obeyed the command and galloped off

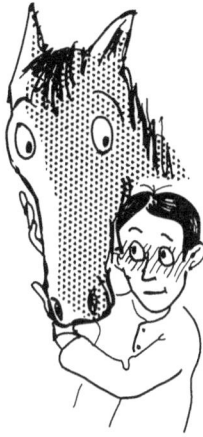

along the familiar road. The thief took off in fright. The young man returned home and spent the remaining hours of darkness with his horse.

In the morning he told his parents what had happened, expressing his anger that anyone should try to steal this precious animal that was almost part of his family.

His father said, "Yes, my son, it is a terrible thing to deprive* another man of his rightful possessions. In this case it is a large and important possession, but even the smallest article should not be disregarded. What is yours is yours, what is mine is mine. No matter how rich or poor you are or I am, there is rarely any excuse for stealing. Sometimes people think it is all right to steal from a group, such as the workers or priests at the temple, or from the market stallholders. They think that in some way those possessions, since they are not individually owned, do not matter so much. But a person's integrity* is damaged in a similar way, should they be a thief of articles belonging to no particular person, or should they be stealing their best friend's donkey."

$\oplus$

Some questions to ask yourself:

? Have you ever had something stolen from you? How did it feel?

? How might you feel about yourself if you dishonestly took something from someone else?

? What effect does shoplifting have on the thief? On the shopkeeper? On other customers? On the price of goods in the shops?

? What would be the result if everyone stole things such as paper, pens and equipment from their place of work or their school?

? What does 'integrity' mean when we think about stealing?

? Can you think of a situation when it might be necessary for someone to steal to stay alive? Could that be wrong too?

STORY 5

Yama 4: Chastity or 'Sexual Self-control' – *Bramacharya*

MY SISTER HAS AN ADMIRER

When my sister, Usha, reached the age of thirteen my mother started to fret about finding her a husband. In India in those days, girls married very young. Life was often short; you had to get on with the business of living before you died.

My sister did not want to think about getting married. She was enjoying being a girl. She enjoyed playing in the rain, swimming in the river and climbing trees.

Mother would scold her saying, "How do you expect anyone to want to marry you when you always look so untidy? Look at your hair; look at the mud on your clothes. You are a young woman now. It's time you stopped all these childish pursuits*!" But my sister did not listen. She was enjoying herself too much!

One day we had a visit from the merchant in the market and his son. They wanted to speak to my father about when our crops would be ready to take to market.

"You must ask my wife about that sort of thing," said my father. "She and my daughter and the servants take care of the crops."

Usha, who was hiding behind the door in the next room, felt herself fill with pride. I saw her straighten up and look important when father mentioned that she was in charge of the crops. She peeped round the corner and her eyes met the eyes of the merchant's son. I have never seen my sister acting as strangely as she did on that morning. She happened to be clean and tidy as it was early in the day and she had not had time to get muddy. She stepped boldly from the shadows and said:

"Father, Mother and I would be very pleased to show Mr Mehta our fields. We can tell him exactly what we have grown and when we hope it will be ready," and she looked across at the young man, a very handsome youth of about sixteen and smiled demurely*.

"Very well, Usha, I'm sure Mother will be very glad of your help," replied Father, and he disappeared, leaving us to show the merchant and his son our crops. I say us, because I certainly did not want to miss out on watching my sister in this new role she had suddenly taken on. It was a transformation*. My sister, instead of laughing, running and skipping, was walking quietly behind my mother who was discussing business with Mr Singh. His son had certainly noticed her. He couldn't take his eyes off her.

My sister asked the young man if he worked in the market with his father.

"Indeed I do, miss," he answered, "but I do not work on Saturdays. Can I come and call on you?"

"I don't know, I'll have to ask my father," said Usha, blushing. She chatted away to the young man about all sorts of things. I soon lost interest and wandered off.

That evening, my sister asked my father at the dinner table if the young man could come to call on her on Saturday. My father stopped eating and looked very serious.

"Ah, my daughter, I see a change is coming to us. I see we need to talk about your future. I have nothing against the young man personally. Indeed he is a fine young man. However, he is not of the same background as you. He is not a *Brahmin**, he is one of the merchant classes, not a high enough caste for this family. If you were to see him and you were to do everything he wanted you to do, you would soon be very close indeed. So close that there would be no space for even a piece of hay to be squeezed between you, then you would have to marry the boy and bring up your child according to his caste*.

"Tell me this, Usha? Do you enjoy the way of life that we have? Do you like to have a big house and land and servants to help you? How would you feel if you lived in a tiny shack and spent most of your time out in the sun working very hard in between rearing your babies with no help at all?"

Usha looked very serious. "I don't think I would like that very much, Father," she said.

"Then why not wait and give yourself properly in marriage to a suitable young man who will provide you with a lifestyle that you are accustomed to. There is plenty of time in spite of what your mother says. She was eighteen when I married her. She refused many suitors* before her perfect man came along..."

My Father looked meaningfully at mother before he turned and left the room.

41

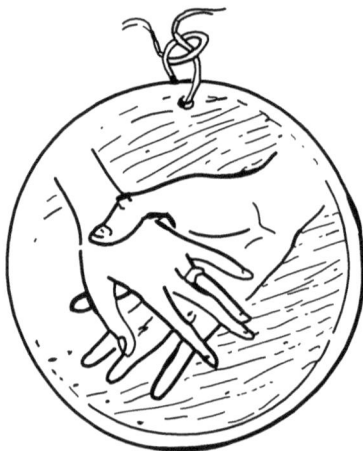

Usha looked downcast.

"What do you think, Mother?" she asked.

"Well, I don't think there's any hurry really, dear. I do agree with Father that it is best to keep your love and your body to yourself until someone suitable in every way comes along. You can be sure that he will. How many unmarried women do you know?"

My sister could not think of any at all.

"Well, my dear, best keep yourself to yourself, stay chaste* rather than be chased, that's what my mother used to say to me! And when a really good suitable hunter comes along, you will be able to enjoy the chase!"

My mother patted Usha. A silence followed. My sister stood up looking wistful*. "Well, I'm off out to climb a tree. You coming Ramu?" she sighed.

"I'm glad you're not going to get married yet," said I. "It's good to have someone to climb trees with. Father says I'm too old to be climbing trees, but I love it!"

⊕

⊕

Note for teachers and yoga students:

This story raises several issues which require some explanation. The caste system is a part of the Indian tradition, where society is divided into different classes or castes. Within each caste people have their own system of values and behaviour. At the top are the *Brahmins*, a class of priests, to which Ramesh and his family belonged. The class below would be the *Kshatriyas*, who in the past were barons and warriors. The *Vaisyas* are the next class, being merchants, or commoners. Next come the *Sudras*, who are the craftsmen and labourers. Below them are those who do very menial work, such as road sweepers. The Hindi name for them is *Harijan*, which means people loved by God – the implication being that nobody else loves them. (*Hari* means Lord, *Jana* means people.) In English they are referred to as 'the Untouchables'.

In the West we have royalty and aristocracy at the top of the social tree, followed by the upper class (landed gentry), then the middle class, and finally the working class. People have resisted the mixing of the classes in general and certainly in the past it would have been frowned upon if, for example, a servant married her master, or if a manservant married the lady of the house.

In India, you are expected to follow your *dharma**, or path in life, according to spiritual law. It is considered taboo* to act against *dharma*. You are expected to marry into your own caste. The word for caste in *Sanskrit** is *vara* and it means 'colour', but has nothing to do with the colour of your skin. It means a leaning towards, a tendency, or an inclination* of the mind.

Hindus believe that we come into this world into an appropriate caste for our required life experience at that time, bearing in mind that they say we each have many lives on this earth. This is the reason it is taboo for people to marry outside their caste. However, a woman may marry a man of one caste above her own, but not a man of a lower caste, because it is thought that she may not respect her husband if he is of a lower caste.

Some modern spiritual leaders now say there is only one caste, the caste of the human race.

Society is gradually becoming more mixed up these days, as education allows those with ability from the lower classes to have good jobs and earn good incomes. In modern times we say that everyone is equal, all human beings are due the same respect.

Usha's father was worried that she might fall in love with a young man who could not provide her with the sort of life that she was used to. This is a practical consideration and a matter of real concern for parents, then as now. In those days (and indeed even now in some areas of countries such as India and Pakistan), families wanted their girls to get married as soon as their periods started, because after that time girls can become pregnant if they have sex. If a married girl became pregnant, she and the child would belong to a family that would be able to support them both emotionally and financially. Although girls in this situation would be very immature, the extended family system would look after the young parents and help them to bring up their children. A girl's mother-in-law would always be available. These days many girls are advised to get an education first, before committing themselves to family life with babies to look after.

⊕

NEW WORDS

Dharma: a person's set path in life

Inclination: leaning towards, preference

Sanskrit: the ancient written language of India

Taboo: forbidden

Some points to consider and questions to ask yourself:

? Your body is precious and you are in control of it. No one has the right to touch it or to persuade you to touch theirs.

? What can you do if people are asking you to do things that might harm your body or put it at risk, or make you embarrassed and ashamed later?

? There is a lot of bad stuff online showing people disrespecting their bodies and allowing other people to do embarrassing or dangerous things. Young people can get the idea that these things are okay and normal. Then they may find themselves in trouble in one way or another if they are persuaded to do those things.

? If you are concerned about anything to do with sex, such as pregnancy, disease, sexting, porn, teenage marriage, ask a wise and trusted adult. There may be a school nurse or counsellor who can help advise you if you cannot ask your parents.

This is a very big and important subject but it is beyond the scope of this book.

STORY 6

Yama 5: Non-greed – *Aparigraha*

First story about greed

YOUNG RAMESH IS TURNED UPSIDE DOWN

One day many years ago, when I was four years old perhaps, our family was sitting around the table and my mother had made some most beautiful sweets. I had never had them before. I tasted one; it was delicious. I looked up to my father and I said: "Daddy, Daddy can I have another one?"

My father looked at me with smiling eyes and he said: "Oh? You weren't happy with the first one? Oh dear, I'll have it back then."

And he turned me upside down.

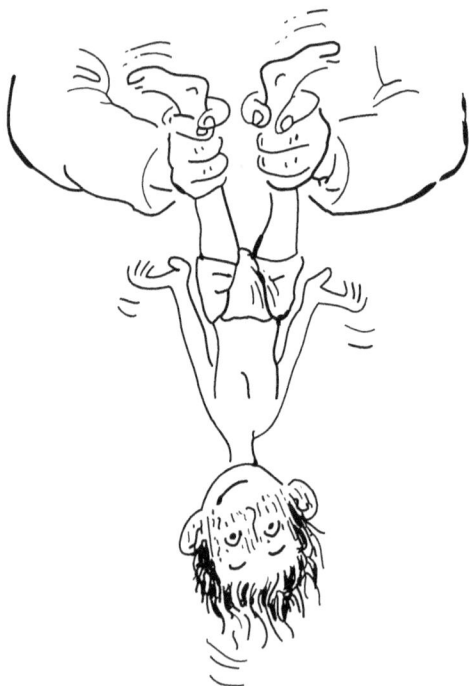

All the family were laughing and smiling at my childish innocence, then he said: "Where is it? Oh! It's gone has it? Never mind, perhaps somebody else would like one now, then maybe if you are very lucky there will be another one left at the end for you."

My father often turned us upside down, just for fun. But this time I remembered it very well, as it came with a message. The message was that

I should only have my share of the food and I should make sure that everyone else has had their share before I ask for more.

$$\oplus$$

Some questions to ask yourself:

? What do you think about sharing food, and not taking more than your 'fair share'?

? Are you tempted to grab as much as you can?

? What do you think of other people who greedily take food, leaving very little for others who are waiting for their share?

STORY 7

Yama 5: Non-greed – *Aparigraha*

Second story about greed

THE MISSING FLOUR

When I was a child we always had plenty of food. The servants too were well fed, but some of them came from families who were not. This was something of a problem for my father. He did not like to think of the brothers and sisters of our servants going hungry. He used to be generous with the sacks of meal that he allowed them to take home. He knew that their families needed help, but the problem did not end there. Each of the families had other contacts – aunts, uncles and in-laws – the number of mouths to feed was apparently infinite, but my father had limited resources*.

In order to be fair and to try to cope with this problem in a way that could be afforded by our household, Father was strict about exactly how many sacks of flour or meal could be distributed amongst the servants' families.

"After all, everyone is related to someone else and I cannot be responsible for feeding the whole neighbourhood!" he would say.

This he made clear to the servants. They nodded their heads in agreement and appeared to understand the situation.

It was my mother's job to keep a record of the number of sacks in the storeroom and to give out the servants' supplies each week. One day she found herself counting the storeroom sacks a second time, and a third. This room was never locked and normally no problems of theft occurred, but on this occasion two sacks of meal were missing. Mother reported the loss to Father on his return from the temple.

"Have you asked the servants where the extra sacks are?" enquired Father.

"No, dear, I thought that if someone had been stealing they would not tell me if I asked."

"We must not assume the worst," replied my father. "Let us go and investigate."

So saying, he and Mother swept off to the storeroom closely followed by my sister Usha and me. This was getting interesting!

"I notice that the ones that are missing are those sacks from the red pile," said Father. "They were the second grade stores. Now where could they be? Let us summon the servants."

We had five people working for us at that time. I had to run and fetch them all from the garden, the cowshed and the kitchen. They all stood in a row outside the food store. Father asked them about the sacks. One of the men began to shuffle his feet. He was a large soft man, recently employed to look after the cattle.

"I can explain, sir, I know where the sacks are. I thought you wouldn't mind, sir, since we take our meals with you. My problem is that I can never eat with the others as I am too busy with the cattle, so I make my own food, sir, and I eat in the cowshed."

"Ah, I remember," said Father. "You were always eating when everyone else had finished. You always had one more *chapati** than everyone else did, and they teased you on account of it. Ramesh told me all about it. Unfortunately he listens to the servants' gossip... So this is how you have solved the problem of your greed? Eating in secret, I see."

The man looked very embarrassed. "I am sorry, sir. I was always hungry as a child. Now when I have food available I feel compelled to eat as much as I can."

The other servants laughed.

"You don't need to do that any more, my friend," said Arundada, the wise old gardener. "In this household you will always have enough. Master is generous. You do not need to be greedy. Give back your flour straight away and think of some jokes to tell us at dinner time. Make sure you wash your hands, though, we don't want the smell of cows to spoil our meal!"

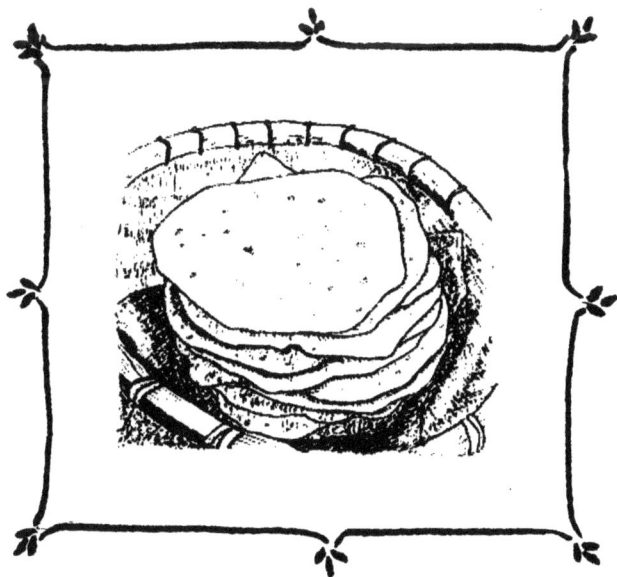

My father smiled and nodded. There was nothing more to say. Over the next few weeks the cowman became less flabby looking and more relaxed. He started to tell jokes and stories and enjoyed his shared meals with the other servants. He had let go of his greed.

⊕

Some questions to ask yourself:

When people are greedy, what happens to:

? their bodies?

? their health?

? their appearance?

? their 'feel-good factor'? (You might call this self-esteem.)

? other people's attitude towards them?

Note that other things can cause people to get fat, for example eating the wrong sort of food, like junk food. Lack of exercise and occasionally illness can also make people too heavy.

STORY 8

Yama 5: Non-greed – *Aparigraha*

Third story about greed – *Aparigraha* also means avarice: an avaricious person is someone who is greedy for possessions

THE AVARICIOUS AUNT

Around the time of my own marriage to Meera, as you can imagine, there was much coming and going. Cousins from many miles away came to stay at my family home. Uncles and aunts whom we had not seen in years appeared and stayed for a few days. When our house was full, my mother arranged for neighbours to put up the extra people.

My marriage was something of a surprise to many people, who had assumed I was to be a monk for the rest of my life. I think they came to see if I had developed cloven* hooves or not.

Although it was quite acceptable to change your life plan, it was somewhat unusual. Some relatives even brought relatives of their own, nothing to do with our family, just to meet me. I think I bore all these meetings with humour and tolerance*, although some of their questions were rather too personal and intrusive* for my liking. There was one particular 'aunt' who was especially curious. She called herself my aunt although neither my father nor mother was related to her.

"How will you adjust to family life now, Ramesh, having had little more than a rice bowl and a robe to your name? I hope you will be able to maintain the good standards of the family," she queried in shrill tones.

I have explained in another story that my branch of the family was less well off when compared to some of the others. This woman came from the branch that had at least fifty servants and a huge estate. She wore gold bangles halfway up her arm and her earrings were so heavy with jewels that they were attached to a band round her head rather than to her ears.

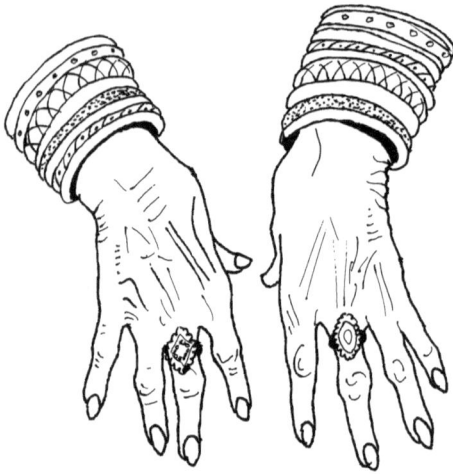

She looked me up and down. "What about your poor wife?" she asked. "How will she manage a home when her husband refuses to have more than one servant? Poor girl, I wouldn't like to be in her shoes."

I smiled and said that Meera and I would be quite contented, thank you very much.

"Contented, hmph!" the aunt squealed. "I personally will never be contented. Contentment does not bring you possessions, servants and jewels. You have to push people. You have to make your demands known and be very firm. You have to be ambitious in your desires for material wealth, never resting until you accumulate* more than you can possibly use. Only then can you rest a little, until the next vision of riches comes to you.

"Then again, throw contentment out of the window and work on that vision. That way you will become truly rich. Everyone will envy you. That is what I long to see, envy on the faces of all I meet. Then I'll know I am worth something. By the way, here is a present for you and Meera when you set up your home." She handed me a little bone tool. I looked up questioningly.

"It's for scraping mud off your boots. I suppose you will be wearing boots sometimes?" she added...

Not only was this woman avaricious, she was also mean-spirited and ungenerous. Of course the two generally go together. As I was debating with myself about how to thank her for the paltry* gift, she swished off in her gold-threaded sari. I watched as she went to harangue* one of the servants about the quality of the ceremonial *chapatis* (flatbreads) that were being served. I was relieved she was not a blood relation of mine...

⊕

Some questions to ask yourself:

? Looking at greed for possessions, such as we see in the West and all over the world in certain sections of society, how do you think people feel when they are never satisfied with the things they have?

? How might it feel to constantly compare yourself to other people who have more than you? Is that a healthy approach to life?

? What signs have you noticed that show you how wasteful we are?

? 'If a whole country is greedy, who goes without?' Think about it. Answers are not simple.

CHAPTER 2

THE *NIYAMAS*

These are known as 'the Observances'. They are the things we should do.

There are five main *Niyamas*:

Niyama 1: Cleanliness or *Saucha* – We should be clean.

Niyama 2: Contentment or *Santosa* – We should be contented.

Niyama 3: Discipline or *Tapas* – We should be disciplined.

Niyama 4: Self-study or *Svadhyaya* – We should learn about ourselves.

Niyama 5: Prayer and meditation, devotion, or *Ishvara Pranidana* – We should meditate or pray.

STORY 9

Niyama 1: Cleanliness – *Saucha*

THE GOLDEN GATES

My father was a very wise man. He used to take us to the riverbank each morning. He would say: "Those who are dirty will never enter the Golden Gates!"

I was very young at the time. I thought he meant the golden gates at the entrance to one of the temples in the town. So one day when I did not want to wash in the river, a holy river it was too, he said to me, "Dirty people will not be allowed through the Golden Gates!"

I told him I did not want to go through the golden gates anyway, because I would only have to wait in the temple for the adults to complete their ceremonies. He said to me that to enter *those* golden gates it was advisable to be clean, but to enter the 'others' (the gates to Heaven) you had to be clean in body, mind and spirit. He wryly* remarked* that since my body was so

64

obviously dirty, it was very possible that my mind and spirit were quite dirty too and needed a good cleansing*.

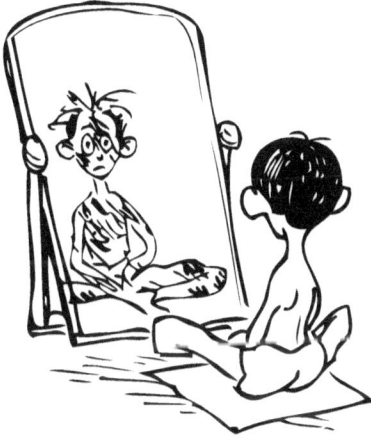

He made a game of washing me thoroughly, so that I was encouraged to do so too. After that he took me along to the temple and made me sit for more than the usual time to 'cleanse* my mind and spirit' also. I was so bored I never complained about washing again!

Some questions to ask yourself:

? Why do you think it is important to keep our bodies clean?

? What did Ramesh's father mean about the 'other' golden gates?

? Our minds can sometimes be troubled with thoughts of hate, jealousy or anger, or other emotions that make us feel bad. Can you think of ways to clear your mind of such thoughts?

? What does 'positive thinking' mean to you?

Niyama 2: Contentment – Santosa

RAMESH AND THE PARROT FEATHERS

When I was a child of about eight my father said to me, "Ramesh, why do you have such a long face?"

He was always aware of my feelings, always observing* and commenting on these things.

"Ramesh, why on this beautiful day, with the birds singing and the river running, do you look sad? What could you have to feel sad about? The world is a beautiful place. Be happy!"

"I cannot be happy today, Father," said I.

"And why is that, my son?"

"Because my brother has more friends than I have. I only have the two boys next door, and he has at least four friends."

"But why should that trouble you, Ramesh? Do you not like your two friends? Are you not completely happy with them when you lose yourselves in the forest, when you climb the trees and wear parrot feathers in your hair?"

"Yes I am happy," I replied, "but maybe I would be even happier with four good friends."

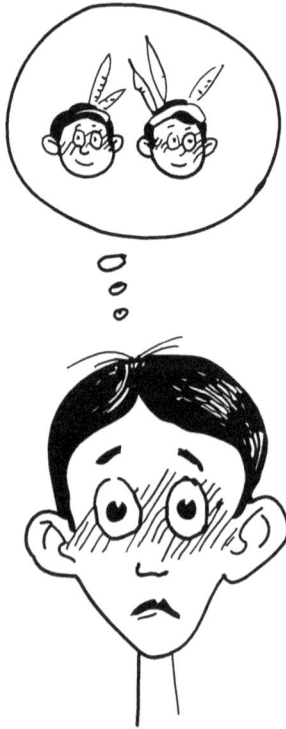

"Happiness is happiness, my son. You cannot measure it. You cannot count it. You must learn to know it when you have it and be content with it, and if you are not lucky enough to be happy one day, then still be content to wait until it comes to you again, for surely it will. God is watching and providing for all of his children, but it makes Him unhappy to see you with a long face. So go and find your friends, my son. You do not want to make God, your father, unhappy do you?"

$\oplus$

NEW WORDS:
Observing: watching carefully

Some questions to ask yourself:

? How do you feel if you always compare yourself to people who have more friends or more possessions than you have?

? How do you feel when you appreciate what you do have and remind yourself about those who are less fortunate?

Not everyone believes in 'God', but it is important to know that our parents or carers like to see us happy and contented, and not always complaining and wanting 'more'.

Niyama 3: Discipline – Tapas

THE STUDENT GETS A THORN IN HIS FOOT

There was once a young man, could it have been me, Ramesh Guptananda? Maybe. This young man decided to follow the path of *Raja yoga**. In truth, he had little idea of the implications of this decision. He found for himself a *guru* who lived in a village some five miles away. To see this man he had to rise well before daybreak and walk the distance, so that the two of them could talk and he could learn and then meditate before the day became too hot.

The first day he set off fired with great enthusiasm and reached the old man as the sun rose. He felt very pleased with himself, very inflated*. The old man looked and smiled at him and spoke encouraging words.

The second day he arrived a little later. The meditation had to be shorter on this occasion, as the sun began to burn up the quiet mind of the student.

On the third day the student got a thorn in his foot so that, already late, he was later than ever.

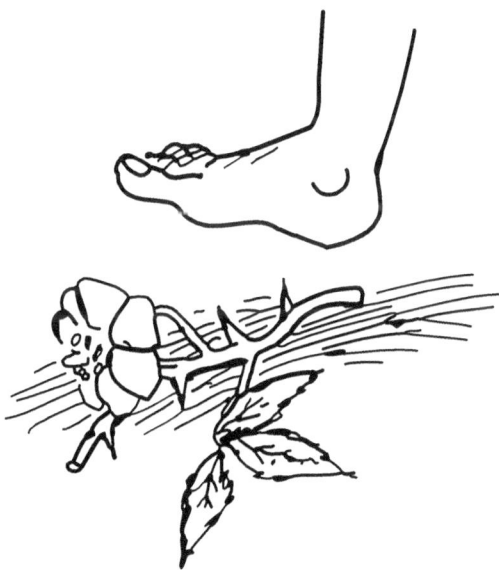

The guru smiled and nodded, then he said, "The Lord will throw down many thorns along your path, my son. Only through discipline, hardening your body and sharpening your mind will you achieve your goal. Thorns are never excuses for failure. The Lord loves you and only does this to prepare you for the difficulties of the world and not to make you suffer for the sake of it. Welcome your hardships and wear your successes quietly on the inside, like jewels adorning* a secret cave. He who waves his medals around for all to see soon has them stolen from him. Tomorrow, arrive before sunrise, and we will pray together and give thanks."

$$\oplus$$

NEW WORDS:

Adorning: decorating

Inflated: puffed up (e.g. with pride)

Raja yoga: a form of yoga intended to achieve control over the mind and emotions

Some questions to ask yourself:

? Ramesh was learning the self-discipline of getting up early in order to achieve his aim of seeing the *guru* before the sun was too hot. What kind of discipline do you need to work on in order to achieve your aims?

? What sort of discipline do you already have in your life?

? How do you feel when there are chaotic, undisciplined people around you?

? How do you feel when you stop behaving in a disciplined manner?

? Can there be too much discipline in people's lives?

? What could be the result of too much discipline?

? 'He who waves his medals around for all to see soon has them stolen from him.' What do you think this means?

STORY 12

Niyama 3: Discipline – *Tapas*

Second story about discipline

THE CHARIOTEER
AND HIS HORSES

The words self-denial*, austerity* and renunciation* are all about giving up worldly pleasures.

You may have noticed that my stories speak of enjoying the gifts of life. They do not encourage denial, although for myself I chose a life of austerity, first as a young man and again later, after my wife had died. In my country we have a tradition of renunciation for those who wish to know God. However, it is well understood that ordinary people, who are not going to become spiritual teachers, have a place for God in their lives. Indeed they too are 'part of God'; we are all divine beings, in exactly the same way as the holy man, the *sanyasin** or the *sadhu**.

They are certainly not to be condemned* for choosing a worldly life. Theirs is the more normal and natural choice. The question arises then, to someone who has not decided to renounce or give up everything worldly, "What should my attitude be towards the pleasures, gifts and talents in and of my life?"

In one of the *Upanishads**, the *Katha** Upanishad*, there is a story that goes like this:

A Lord is in his chariot. The question is, does he have control of his horses, or are they badly trained or wild? Is he a good horseman, or a bad one? If he has trained his horses well he will reach his goal. If he has not he will be pulled hither and thither, the horses ever seeking greener pastures.

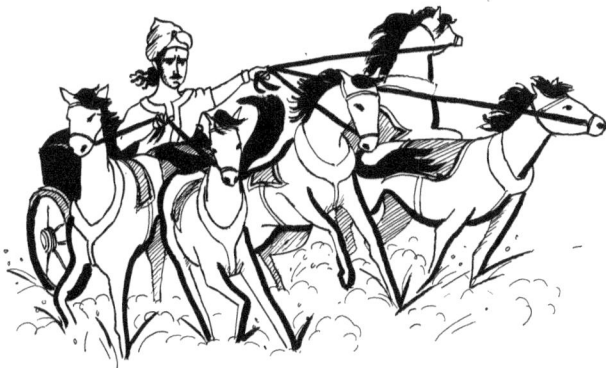

This is a parable (simple story) to show us what we human beings are like. The Lord is the Self, or the person, and the chariot is their body. The five horses are the five senses. The reins are the mind that controls the senses. If the mind is disciplined, the senses are under control and the Self reaches the desired destination. An undisciplined approach results in these 'wild horses' leading the person to seek to gratify or please their senses all the time. They want to smell, touch, taste, see and hear beautiful things as much as possible, and then they find they are out of control.

We have our senses in order to appreciate our surroundings and to help us to survive in the environment. They do a very good job. With regard to survival, the smell of burning immediately causes alarm bells to ring in our minds.

With regard to enjoying our world, the joy of seeing and smelling a beautiful rose is well worth experiencing. The pleasure of eating a carefully prepared meal is well worth waiting for. The delight of feeling a lover's touch, to see their face, to smell their perfume, to taste their lips, is quite exquisite. The problem lies in what occurs when we are constantly thinking about gratifying our senses, to the exclusion of almost everything else.

This is a very common state of mind in many people. They are never satisfied. No sooner have they pleased themselves in one way than they are looking to gratify themselves in another. Their horses are wild; the charioteer is not in control of the chariot, which lurches this way and that, chasing after experiences of the senses.

The soul is bewildered*, something is missing from their life and they do not understand what it is. They begin to wonder if they should give up everything and become a monk or a nun. These desires are driving them crazy or making them sick. There is nothing deep or substantial* about their life, which is being lived on the surface of things.

Finally, their chariot breaks down and their body becomes ill. There are, of course, other reasons for a body becoming ill, but sense gratification is a very common one. People become diabetic, or get liver disease or lung cancer or a multitude of other complaints. Only then are they forced to take stock* of the situation.

This is a sad state of affairs. If only they had applied some moderation. If only they had shown some consideration for their poor chariot. The disciplined charioteer understands that their horses need to be controlled. Sometimes they may be allowed to have full rein, but not every day, and not all the time, because they will soon run out of energy.

After the race, the resting period, the quiet time, abstinence*, reflection, and the building of strength for other purposes are needed. These other purposes will include your *dharma*, or duty in life. Duty can be towards yourself and is certainly towards other people as well. When we are constantly running a wild chariot race of self-gratification*, how can we be thinking about the needs of others in our life? We may have parents, brothers, sisters, a partner, and friends, all of whom are important to us and need our time and attention, just as we need theirs at times. A disciplined person has enough time for themselves and enough time for other people in their life.

$\oplus$

NEW WORDS:

Abstinence: When a person chooses not to satisfy their appetites, e.g. for certain foods, drugs, alcohol or sexual activities

Austerity: being very stern or serious

Bewildered: confused or puzzled

Condemned: said to be wrong

***Katha*:** The *Katha Upanishad* is a selection of Hindu verses in which freedom from desire is discussed

Renunciation: giving up or rejecting something, e.g. worldly pleasures, family life

***Sadhu*:** a Hindu monk

***Sanyasin*:** a Hindu holy man

Self-denial: saying 'No', or refusing to enjoy the material pleasures of life, e.g. money, fashion, married life, extravagant food

Self-gratification: pleasing the senses or satisfying your own desires

Substantial: solid, concrete or serious

Take stock: to consider, assess

***Upanishads*:** a collection of very old religious texts from India

Niyama 4: Self-study – Svadhyaya

RAMESH LEARNS MORE ABOUT HIMSELF

When I was a teenager of about fourteen, my father told me that I was far too selfish. He told me to go to the market for Mother to purchase several herbs and spices, which he then named. I told him I would not recognise all of them.

"You have been eating food in this house for fourteen years, and you do not know which herbs your mother uses?" he said, raising his eyebrows. "Go to the market and ask Mala, who sells all the condiments*, to show you what is what. She knows your mother well and would not deceive you."

So I went to market and found the old woman.

"Ah, it is you, Ramesh," said she, and when I explained the problem she laughed and told me I was unfamiliar with the very things that had been keeping me well and strong all these years.

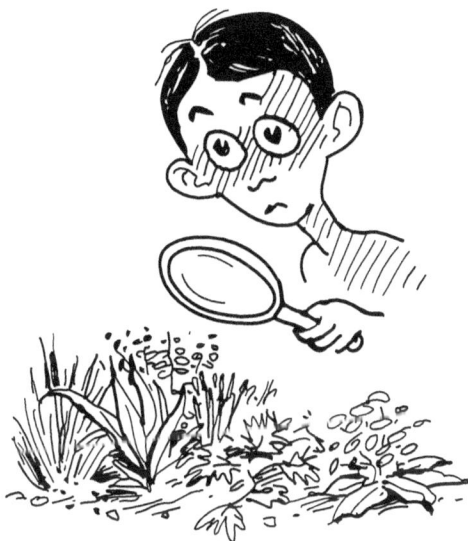

"But it does not surprise me," she said. "Children pay little attention to 'what' and 'why', but, like the plants, they just grow. You must learn what keeps you well, Ramesh, and what makes you ill. You must learn what makes you happy and what sad. You need to know these things for yourself so that you can regulate* your own life. You cannot rely on the knowledge of others for this information. You travel alone in this world. You truly only have yourself. Sometimes you will indeed be alone – no partner, no parents to help you. Look at yourself; ask questions of the Lord God in your meditations. Know yourself. Only then will you be able to understand and help others."

$$\oplus$$

NEW WORDS:

Condiments: the kinds of food that flavour a dish, e.g. salt, pepper, herbs, spices

Regulate: to control by rules

Some questions to ask yourself:

? What keeps me healthy?

? What do I enjoy doing?

? What am I good at?

? How can I develop myself, my gifts, talents and abilities?

Niyama 5: Devotion
– Ishvara Pranidana

This could be understood as prayer
and meditation

THE SPECIAL BREAD

When I was a child of fourteen, my family used to visit the temple regularly. We would bring offerings of food with us. In our eyes it was food for God, but my father explained that God would not want it to be wasted, as he had no need for actual food. The staff and the families of the temple workers and the poor of the town would use our fruit and bread.

One day my mother baked some bread and put some delicious flavourings into part of the batch. I was disappointed to find that the most flavoursome loaves were to be taken to the temple especially for the ceremony to honour the great god *Shiva**. I complained. My father overheard my complaint.

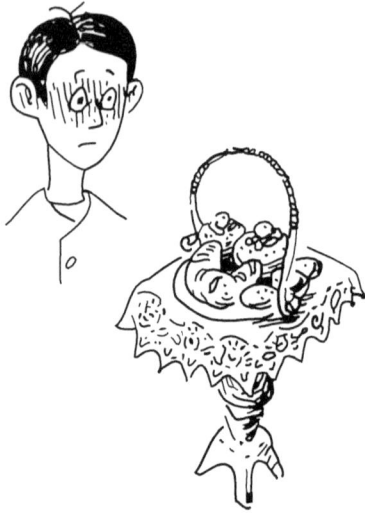

"I do understand that boys of your age think of little else than their stomachs," said he, "but I would like you to remember this! Remember that everything you eat comes by the grace of God. Remember that it is by the grace of God that you are alive today and that it was not you, but poor Kumar, who was thrown off the ox and trampled. Remember that, by the grace of God, your sister recovered from her illness last year. Her sight was restored to her after we took her to the temple and the priests laid their hands upon her and prayed. No, my son, you must not resent these meagre* gifts which we take to Lord

Shiva*, who has been kind to our family. He has provided everything for us. He has not used his powers of destruction on us; we have been spared.

Remember, my son, when your belly calls for more food and looks hungrily at the sacrifice we have made to the Lord, that we must show our gratitude to the Lord because He loves us. The least we can do is to love Him back. He likes to hear our prayers and to see our unselfish acts. He wants us to feed the poor and the hungry and the workers at the temple because He has fed us."

I felt very small by this time. My father did not have to remind me ever again. I was indeed grateful for my good life, my healthy family and our good fortune.

$\oplus$

NEW WORDS:

Meagre: poor, small, not enough

Shiva: the great Hindu god of destruction and reproduction, or breaking down and building up

Some thoughts:

We should consider that there may be help and guidance available through prayer and meditation. If you believe in God then you should pray.

? For those who believe in God from whatever religion, this story will make sense.

? Those who have no belief in God might like to think of serving or helping their fellow human beings as most important. If we all take care of each other we will not go far wrong.

? We all have a duty to feed the poor and to look after those who give their lives to helping others, such as the temple workers in this case.

CHAPTER 3

THE LESS WELL-KNOWN *YAMAS* AND *NIYAMAS*

STORY 15

Tolerance, Forgiveness and Understanding

THE ANGRY YOUNG MAN

When I was a youth, I was not known for my tolerance*. Everyone seemed to irritate me at times. My mother was constantly reminding me to do this and that. My father would always want to know what I was going to be doing, not just that day, but next week and even next month! My sister was always asking questions.

My irritation grew and grew until it was difficult for my family to speak to me without me beginning to burn up inside. I did not, however, tell them what I was feeling, because I realised that it was not right. In fact, it was not just them, I was in the wrong too, but somehow this knowledge did not help me to get over the problem.

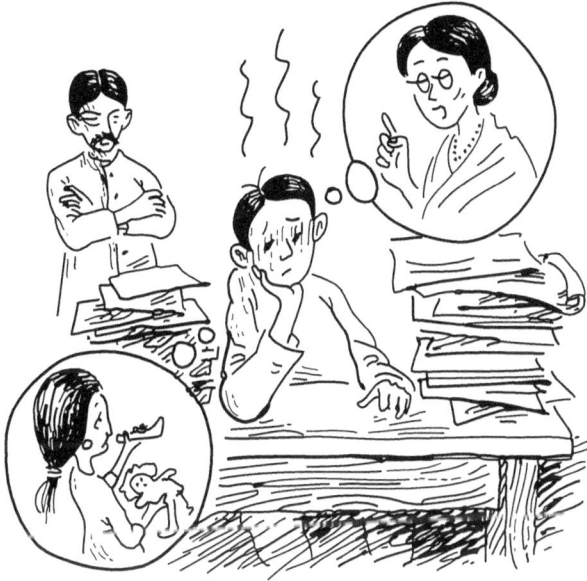

One day, I was finishing some work which my father had given me to do, when my sister came along and started to ask me all about it. Now, I had not enjoyed the work and just wanted to forget about it. I said something dismissive* and walked out. My sister chased after me saying, "Ramu, why won't you talk to me? I like talking to you but you don't answer my questions these days. How am I going to learn if no one answers my questions?" Then she burst into tears and ran off.

When I went indoors for my evening meal,

my mother started to say to me, "Ramu, have you cleaned out the stable today? I noticed that you didn't do it yesterday; and did you remember to give your washing to Gopika? And..."

I walked out; I could not take any more, but there, outside, was my father.

"Ah, Ramesh, what do you plan to do next week, after you have finished the work you started today? I had in mind some illuminated[*] prayers which you could work on, to present at the temple in time for the festival."

I did not turn my back on my father, that would have been unthinkable, but I stood there saying nothing and fuming. All these people were demanding things of me all the time. I just wanted them to leave me alone to make decisions for myself for a change. My father noticed my discomfiture[*].

"Ah, Ramesh, I see you are struck dumb[*]. What is the problem?"

I just couldn't tell him. I felt so irritated and did not understand why. I heard myself saying, "Everybody wants me to do things all the time. I get no peace at all!"

"Now, Ramesh, you know that is not true, for most of the day you have been left alone to get on with your work."

"But it was not my work, it was what you wanted me to do and I felt as if you were there watching me all the time."

"It is indeed difficult to reconcile* yourself with the need to work and to do all the things which need to be done, when someone else always seems to notice what needs to be done before you do," my father replied. "But that is the nature of things, you know. Your mother will always notice things you should do, often before you do. It is because she is used to that way of thinking – she has been doing it for years. I too can foresee what has to be done. What I am trying to do for you is to show you how to plan ahead for yourself, so that I can actually take a rest and sit back and watch you unfold your future in a useful and constructive* way."

"Oh, now I understand, Father," said I. "Sometimes I have been thinking you don't trust me to get anything done on my own!"

"Be tolerant of your parents' guidance, my son," said my father. "Take it in the spirit in which it is meant. Perhaps we have pushed you too far on occasions, but you could quietly remind us of the fact and, if we see you remembering to do things of your own accord, we will certainly loosen the reins. Let us keep the channels of communication open. Do not let your intolerance drive a wedge between us. Give us your forbearance* and we will continue to give you our forgiveness for all the things you have omitted to do, but will not admit to!"

Then he smiled and patted me on the shoulder. At that moment I remembered I had not given my saddle to the mender the previous day, as I had promised Father I would do. I looked at my father to see if he was going to check on that too. He winked at me as if he could read my mind and said, "Come along, son, let us eat." We went in together to join my sister and my mother. My anger had evaporated.

$\oplus$

NEW WORDS:

Constructive: valuable, practical, beneficial

Discomfiture: being worried, anxious or confused

Dismissive: sending away, not giving consideration to what is being said

Forbear/Forbearance: to 'put up with' patiently

Illuminated: illustrated, having pictures

Intolerant: not being able to bear or to put up with other people's opinions and actions

Reconcile: to adjust

Struck dumb: without a voice

Tolerance: being willing to accept other people's opinions and actions

Some questions to ask yourself:

? Can you think of anyone you are intolerant towards at times?

? What is it about them that you don't like?

? Is anyone intolerant towards you?

? How does it feel?

? Do you try to understand others?

? How does it feel to forgive someone?

? How does it feel to be forgiven?

STORY 16

Endurance*, Forbearance* and Obedience*

ARUN USES HIS IMAGINATION

Sometimes old Arundada* the gardener would sit back after his meal and tell us children stories. I always listened avidly*, as he seemed to have had an interesting life, very different from our world of home, temple and market.

When he was a young man he worked on ships. He had a lot of physical work to do and not much to eat at the end of the day. He would be sent up on the rigging and down into the hold. He would survive on little more than a bowl of rice each day. It was very surprising to us that he did what he did and stayed healthy and alive.

Arundada said that he used to pray a lot and ask for God's help when he was feeling tired and hungry. He used to make his meagre* bowl of rice last as long as possible and would imagine while he was eating it that it was actually a delicious stew of beans and vegetables. He would chew it over and over until he could not feel any texture in it at all, before he swallowed it. He would keep his eyes shut while he ate and imagine he was in a beautiful place by the sea, sitting under a palm tree and enjoying a feast in the warm sun. He would allow the goodness of the food to permeate* his skinny body and feel the warmth emanating* from it.

He would always try to sit in the sun in the cool of the evening while he ate. He wanted to absorb the warmth of the sun's rays. He said he was always thankful for his food, even though it was very meagre*, because he realised that many people had less to eat than he had.

Once, after a particularly hard day's work, he was sitting under his imaginary palm tree, munching away at his rice. On this occasion, he told himself that it was a beautiful salad of fruit and nuts.

A large heavy object came falling towards him. He jumped out of his reverie*. The object had been thrown by one of his companions who had always envied Arun his tranquillity*. He had himself constantly railed* against all the

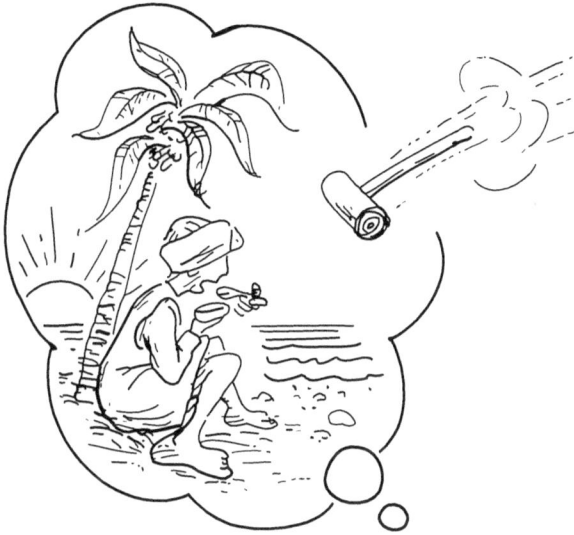

restrictions* of the life that had been imposed on him, as he saw it. He would far rather not be working on a ship. He would rather be travelling the land on horseback, meeting new people and seeing new sights. But this was not to be: he had lost his horse and most of his possessions and had been obliged to join the ship. He had found himself growing thinner and thinner until the bones in his body seemed to press through the flesh, while Arun still glowed with health.

Arun looked up. "What is it, Vijay? What is troubling you this time?"

"You! There you sit with your eyes closed peacefully eating and getting fat while the rest of us starve. I hate you, you smug idiot!"

"Why do you let your hate and fear spoil your life, my friend?" Arun asked. "Why not adjust your viewpoint? Take another look at your life. You will survive much better if you let go of your anger. It is burning you up. Thank God for what you do have. Do not be angry about what you don't have. You are always angry when the captain and the first mate tell you what to do. Why? That is their place on this ship. They are doing what they are supposed to do. If you obey the orders that they rightfully give you without question, you will be happier and so will they. You will be at peace, so will they. The atmosphere between you will change. You may discover that they are only human beings like yourself. Let go of your resentment* and your bitterness, my friend, and life will go more smoothly for you."

Arundada told me that eventually this man became his friend and wanted to know all about his palm tree. He learned to meditate and began to grow healthy again. He was a changed man when at last the ship returned to land.

⊕

NEW WORDS:

Arundada: Grandfather Arun

Avidly: keenly

Consequences: results

Emanating: coming from

Endure/endurance: withstand, bear up against, survive

Forbear/forbearance: put up with patiently

Meagre: scant, poor, not enough

Obedience: doing what you are told

Permeate: spread through

Railed: complained bitterly

Resentment: displeasure, bitterness, anger

Restrictions: things that prevent people from doing what they want to do

Reverie: daydream

Tranquility: calmness, peacefulness, serenity

Some questions to ask yourself:

? What have you learned to endure[*]?

? How has that helped you?

? Does anyone show forbearance[*] towards you? In other words do they put up with your bad habits willingly?

? What would it be like in school if there were no rules, or if nobody obeyed the rules?

? What are the dangers of blind obedience[*] – obeying without thought about the consequences[*]?

Sincerity* and Earnest* Endeavour*

ANIL IS AT HOME ON THE FARM

You may have been wondering about my brother and why he does not feature much in my stories. It is because he went to live with my uncle quite early on in his life, as my uncle and aunt had no children of their own. This made Uncle Sanjay and his wife very distraught*. My mother and father knew that my brother, Anil, was very fond of Uncle and Aunt and that he would be happy with them. Initially* he was told nothing about the plan, but went to stay with them for a short holiday. My uncle kept many animals and this was a lifestyle my brother enjoyed greatly. Not for him the goings on at the temple; he would rather be riding horses. When he returned, after two weeks, he talked non-stop about Uncle's place.

"Did you enjoy it so much that you cannot

think of anything else, my son?" asked my mother.

"I wish we had a farm," said Anil wistfully*.

"How about if you went to stay with Uncle for longer to see if you really prefer that kind of life?"

My brother's eyes lit up. "Could I really? Could I go and stay with Uncle all the time and come here for holidays?" he asked.

"What if you get lonely and start to miss your brother Ramesh, and your sister? What if you miss us, your parents?"

"Oh, yes, I know I will miss you, but I know that I am a lot of help to my uncle and my aunt says he is never happier than when I am with him. She says they are very sad not to have their own son and I could be like a son to them. I would still love you all of course!" said he, looking apologetically* round at the family.

My sister and brother were not very close. They used to squabble* quite a lot; my sister wanted to have my brother's bedroom, but he would never agree to move out of it. She sat quietly, not saying a word during this conversation. She did not want it to seem as though she wanted him to go, but secretly she was quite happy about it.

It was decided that my brother should live with our uncle for a trial period of six months to see if we were all happy with the new situation. He would be able to visit us regularly, as my uncle would bring his produce to market most weeks.

During that six months, my brother showed himself to be a true farmer, especially with the animals. He loved and cared for them; he cleaned them out and bathed their wounds. He worked very hard to show that he would be a worthy addition to their family.

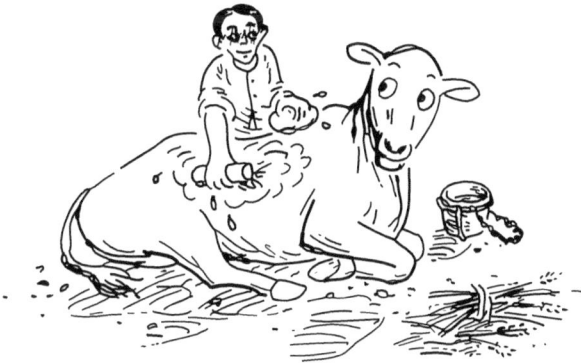

One day, when he and my uncle called to see us, Uncle Sanjay said, "Young Anil here is the best worker I've had in a long time. Trouble is, he doesn't know when to stop. We call him in for his meals and he says he isn't hungry, he's too busy with the cattle!"

My brother looked down at his feet.

"You'll learn," said my father. "Earnest* endeavour* is one thing, but you must not become addicted to work. We all need time to enjoy ourselves."

"But work is my enjoyment!" protested Anil.

"Well, I'm not really complaining," said Uncle. "When I said he's the best worker I've had in a long time, I meant it sincerely*. I could not wish for a better nephew, or are you my son now, Anil?"

We all laughed and my father said, "Well, let's look at his ears. No, I think he's still my son. Only my family have ears that stick out like that!"

⊕

NEW WORDS:

Apologetically: wanting to say he was sorry

Distraught: anxiously worried, distracted

Earnest: serious, purposeful

Endeavour: try hard, work

Initially: at first

Squabble: argue over small things

Sincerely, sincerity: (with) genuine honesty

Wistful: a vague longing

Some questions to ask yourself:

? How do you feel when somebody promises to do something for you and does not do it?

? Do you ever make promises you know you can't keep?

? How do you feel after making a real effort with some work, compared to times when you didn't really bother much?

STORY 18

Compassion* and Sympathy

AUNT USHMA BECOMES VERY ILL

When I was a small child I had an aunt, she was my mother's sister. She used to live with us and help my mother look after us children. She would wash us and rock us to sleep if we were unsettled. She was always available to help in any way and never asked for anything in return. My mother used to say to us, "You must look after your Auntie Ushma as well as she looks after you!"

A time came when we did indeed have to carry out our mother's wishes. Aunt Ushma became very ill. All she could do was lie in bed and drink water and sometimes a little fruit juice. Everyone was very worried about her. I used to like to go and visit her and stroke her hair as it lay on the pillow beside her. She would turn her head and smile a wan* smile.

"Ah, Ramu," she would say, "how nice it is to feel your cool hands on my forehead. No one has hands like yours. I am sure you will be a great healer one day."

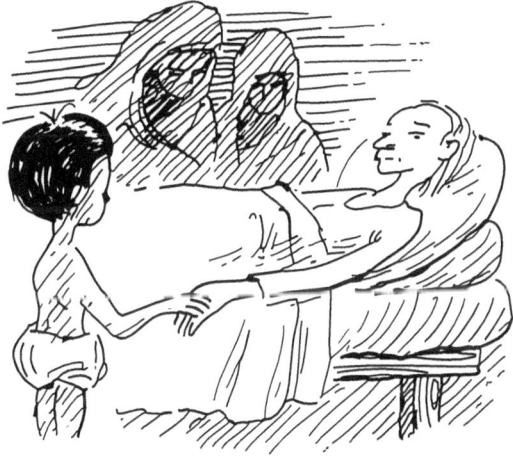

Well, I didn't know what she was talking about. I just knew I wanted her to get well again quickly, so that we could enjoy our usual pursuits*, our walks along the riverbank and playing hide-and-seek in the woods. She was ill for a long time, it seemed to me. She grew so thin that her skin looked like paper drawn across the bones of her face. No one could help her. The priest visited her and so did the wise woman who sold the herbs in the market. The *guru* who lived in the nearby mountain was summoned*, but he refused to come. Instead he promised to pray for her each day until he had news of a change for the better. Finally, after several months of illness, Aunt Ushma died. On her last day, she asked to see the family all together. She addressed us all, saying:

"I am going home soon, do not weep for me. I will return as indeed we all do. I hope my next life will shine with a few more jewels than this one. However, in this life I have been blessed with a good number of jewels until recently. I would like to thank you, all of you, for your kindness to me during this tiresome illness. You could not have looked after me with more care or consideration than if I had been the goddess *Shakti** herself." With that she closed her eyes and fell asleep. She never uttered another word. She died during the night.

I always remembered what she had said about my hands, and if members of the family were ill, I made sure I was there to stroke their brows and hold their hands. They always appreciated it, and in later years I did indeed find that my healing gift was called upon by many.

⊕

NEW WORDS:

Compassion/compassionate: kindness, kind-hearted, understanding

Pursuits: activities

Shakti: Hindu Goddess, the Great Divine Mother

Summoned: ordered to come

Unsympathetic: not understanding or kind

Wan: weak, pale, ill-looking

Some questions to ask yourself:

? What do you think Aunt Ushma meant when she spoke about the 'jewels' in her life?

? What kind of effect does an understanding smile have on you?

? Think of a time when you felt compassionate towards someone. How did you show it?

? When someone is unsympathetic* towards you, how do you feel about them?

? A friend is looking for sympathy, but you wonder if they are just being silly. How could

you deal with that and show you are still a
good friend?

Penance* and Retribution* for Wrongdoing

THE MAD MULE

In my town there was a family, Kumar by name, who never seemed to be acceptable to the rest of society. The various members were always in trouble. One would steal a horse; another would do a bad deal with some grain and then later sell some sick animals to an unsuspecting* buyer. The local people got to know their unsavoury* ways, but visitors and travellers were easy prey for them.

On one occasion, a party of travellers was passing through and they required a mule to replace theirs, which had become lame during their journey. Unfortunately for them, the first person they spoke to about obtaining a replacement mule was 'Big Kumar', as he was known. He had several mules that he was trying to sell. One in particular looked like a very healthy beast, as indeed he was, but he had a terrible temper. He was almost a legend in his own lifetime. He had kicked his owner on numerous occasions and broken carts by running off with them. He had even killed a child who ran into his path one day as he was galloping wildly down the road, having broken free from his tether.

Now Big Kumar wondered how he could persuade the travelling family to pay a good price and take this 'Devil mule' off his hands. After much thought he came up with a plan. He would drug the animal with soporific* herbs that were given to people suffering from anxiety. This, he thought, would be a good way of solving his problem.

The unsuspecting visitors were duly taken to view the beast the day before they planned to continue their journey. The 'Devil' had been well fed with the special herbs that calm and steady. He looked good; he was quiet and he even let the buyer ride him down the road and back. The man was delighted. He paid over the asking price and led the beast away. Now Big Kumar knew that the effect of the herbs would wear off by the next day, so he followed the visitor to discover where the mule was to be stabled.

He returned in the night to dose the 'Devil' with more herbs and, thinking that the visitors would soon be on their way, he forgot all about them.

Two days later, a deputation* arrived at his stall in the market. It was the new owner of the 'Devil' walking with a crutch, his wife with a broken arm and his daughter with her fingers bandaged up. With them were a priest and the local magistrate*. It transpired* that the travellers had put off their departure to attend a local feast and, while they were away celebrating, the mule had broken loose.

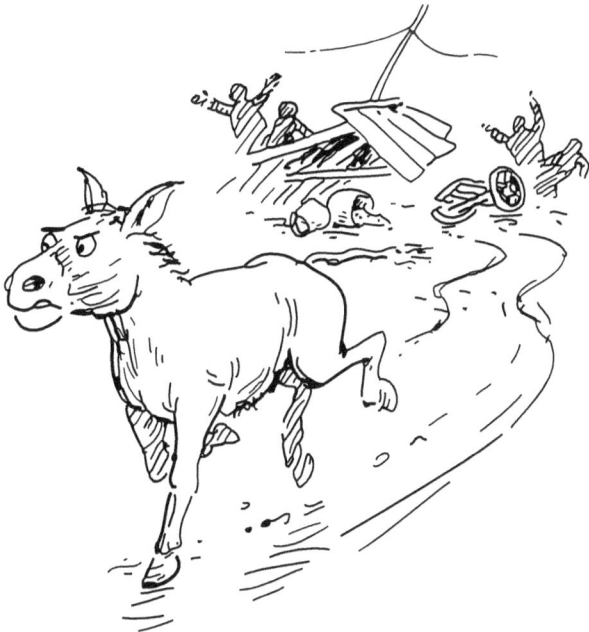

He had charged down the road, sending people and animals flying in all directions, until he had come to an open area of grazing land. The visitors had sustained their injuries while trying to capture him. They had come to demand their money back from Big Kumar. The priest and the magistrate were there to back them up. The magistrate spoke sternly:

"Not only will you return all the money you have received in payment for this terrible animal, but you will have to pay a penance* for trying to convince these good people that this was a usable mule. You are required to spend the whole of next month cleaning the latrines* at the temple and in addition this mule must be slaughtered*."

No matter how much Big Kumar protested, he was obliged to pay for his misdeeds. He would always think twice before cheating the visitors after his embarrassment over the mad mule.

⊕

NEW WORDS:

Deputation: a group of people gathered to represent someone who is complaining

Latrines: toilets used by many people

Magistrate: a judge

Penance: a penalty, something you do to make up for wrongdoing

Retribution: punishment that happens as a result of wrongdoing

Slaughtered: killed

Soporific: causing sleep or drowsiness

Transpired: came to light, became known

Unsavoury: unpleasant, distasteful

Unsuspecting: trusting

Some questions to ask yourself:

? Imagine that you have been thoughtless and inconsiderate, we all are sometimes. You have upset people. What would be the best way to make everyone, including yourself, feel better about it?

? What does 'make the punishment fit the crime' mean?

? A young criminal may have to do community service, working for no pay, rather than go to prison to pay for his crimes. Why might that be better option?

STORY 20

Faith

RAMESH REBELS

This is a story about me, Ramesh Guptananda, when I was a youth, questioning everything that my parents held dear. I did not necessarily want to do what they indicated would be a suitable career for me. I had my doubts about all the activities centred on the temple. I saw people attending ceremonies and then the same people would lie and cheat each other when it came to buying and selling goods. I began to wonder if they were all hypocrites* and if they only attended at temple to show the rest of the world that they were God-fearing souls and could be trusted in business and in their other dealings with people.

One day, when I was feeling particularly antagonistic* to the idea of attending a ceremony to *Lord Rama**, I told my mother that my clothes were dirty and that I could not go.

"Well, you must borrow something from your father's wardrobe then," said she.

I found another excuse. "I have to exercise Raja this afternoon. I couldn't take him out yesterday and he needs a run."

"You could do that this morning," said Mother.

Finally I told her how I was really feeling about the ceremonies and about my doubts as to the gods' existence, or at least as to the nature of God. I felt that if the gods or God did exist, he surely would not want hypocrites, liars and thieves amongst his congregation.

"Ramu," said mother, with a sad look in her eye. "It is true that we are all weak human beings – some of us are weaker than others. You for example…"

I looked at her intently. What was she going to accuse me of now?

"You know the difference between right and wrong: there is no possibility of you stealing your neighbour's horse, or hay from his stable. But someone less well informed than you might be tempted to do this. Then, even if they weren't discovered by their victims, God would know what they had done and they would be diminished* by their crime.

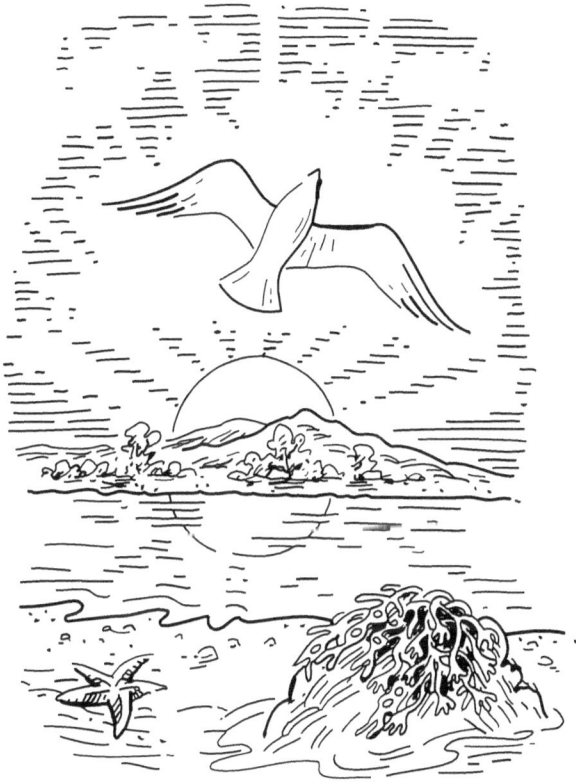

"It is not right to turn away from God just because some of his subjects are not as well brought up as you were. That does not make sense. Is your faith so weak that you feel that you can neglect the Almighty* just because of a few rough types? You need to pray to God. He answers prayers. If you do not pray he may leave you to get on with your life all by yourself. How would that feel? You know that God has answered our prayers on many occasions. So, my son, stiffen your sinews*, work on your resolution which you made two years ago to serve the Lord in every way that you can. Just go to the ceremony this afternoon. He is not asking you to give up your life in his service is he? Off you go. Take Raja out now and wear your father's clothes this afternoon."

I went out. It was a beautiful day and the perfume of the flowers was intoxicating*. The reflection of the sun sparkled on the holy river. I realised that I could not possibly exist without thanking the Lord at the very least, each time I enjoyed His beauty and His bounty*.

I went to the ceremony that afternoon, and in my meditations I was shown a great light, which seemed to start in the distance and get closer and closer until it finally enveloped* me and filled me with a sense of love and peace. My faith came back to me without a shadow of a doubt. God was all around us, inside us and outside us. I was part of God and God was part of me. And I knew.

☩

NEW WORDS:

Almighty (the): God

Antagonistic: against, not wanting to

Bounty: the wonderful gifts of nature

Diminished: to be made smaller/lesser

Enveloped: wrapped, surrounded

Hypocrite: a person who pretends to be what he or she is not

Intoxicating: absolutely delightful, something which makes you feel drunk

Lord Rama: a major god in the Hindu religion

Overarches/overarched: includes/d, encompasses/d

Resolve: firm decision

Stiffen your sinews: become strong

Some questions to ask yourself:

? How does it feel to have faith in someone – to know that they are always to be trusted and will always treat you fairly?

? Can people have faith in you in the same way?

? Ramesh's family had faith in their Hindu gods, and in the Great God Brahma, whom they believed 'overarched'* all the others. Faith comes by way of family tradition, or through the study of spiritual matters. It comes very easily to some people, while others struggle with it or reject it. What different faiths have you heard about, e.g. Christian, Muslim?

? People who believe in God are called believers, those who do not know whether there is a God and an 'afterlife' are known as agnostics, and atheists do not believe in God at all. What do you think about faith in God at this time in your life?

Charity and Non-gossip

RAJA GETS SOAKED

One day, my family was preparing for a feast at the temple. My mother was concerned about what we would all wear and about all the food that she needed to prepare. My father was trying to keep her calm, offering to take on any responsibilities, which she could offload onto him. My sister and I were very excited and kept jumping up and down, running hither and thither and generally getting in the way.

The day was fine as usual, but the rainy season was about to start. The air had a slightly different smell to it. My father announced that he would be preparing for the rains that day and that, if my mother needed him, she should call. Mother continued with her work. She gave me a little job to do and asked my sister to help with the baking. The servants were all very busy too, as they also would attend this feast.

My father reappeared to announce that there was a hole in the stable roof and that if we did not mend it today, Raja, my horse, might get a soaking. No one seemed to be available to help, so I went along to give Father a hand. We gathered the necessary materials and tools and started our work. I had to hold things steady while my father did the fixing. He was not very good at this sort of work, because normally the servants would do it, but on this day no one was free and the rain was imminent*. It had to be done. Finally we finished. I thought the roof might still leak a little, but I said nothing as it had taken us a very long time to complete the work.

Shortly after midday a rumble was heard in the distance. The rain clouds had gathered and were about to burst. I ran into the stable to stand under the mended hole with Raja. We looked up as the first large drops hit the roof. Soon there was a downpour. It was torrential*. You forget how hard it can rain when you've had several months with no rain at all.

At first, the mend held fast, but so relentless* was the torrent, that first a trickle, then a stream of water began to emerge from the hole. I was furious. What would my lovely horse do? He would get wet and he would have a pool of water in his bed. I pulled up my jacket over my head – my smart new jacket donned* for the celebrations – and I ran outside. I was so cross I just wanted to find my father to shout at him and tell him what I thought of his mending skills.

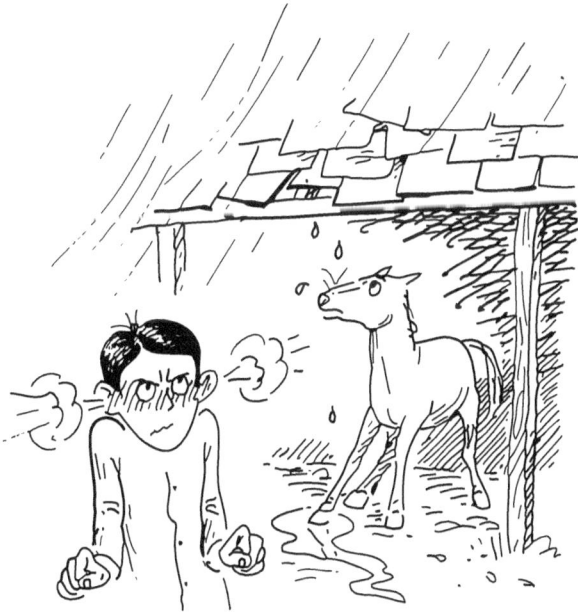

On the way to the house I saw Arundada, the gardener – he was the one who would usually do such work. I told him my father had made a terrible job of mending the hole in the roof and that he would have to fix it immediately, or my horse might catch a cold and die. I ran back indoors, and there was my father, warm, dry and smiling.

"Father!" I shouted. "That mend was useless. Poor Raja is soaking wet and he has a huge puddle to lie in! You're not much good at mending roofs, are you?"

"Well, well, Ramesh, I see you are a little overwrought*. It is not the end of the world that the roof has leaked. Maybe the gardener would have made a better job of it than I did, but at least I made an effort. Can the gardener read as well as I can? Does he know as many prayers as I do? I doubt it, but I do not insult him for that. He does his work and I do mine, generally speaking. Be charitable* towards your poor father, who has tried to do his best. Give me credit for making an effort at least."

"I am sorry, Father," said I and, realising my haste, I blushed. "I told him you were useless at mending things. I should not have said that."

"Well, well, if they gossip about me at least it will only be about my lack of ability to mend the roof and not about a more serious transgression*. But I don't think Arundada has

126

a harsh word to say about anybody. I think my secret is safe with him, don't you?"

The rain had stopped when we went out again and had another try at mending the roof. Even so, Arundada still had to come and fix it the next day. Neither Father nor I were very good at mending roofs!

⊕

NEW WORDS:

Charitable: kind, considerate, generous

Donned: put on

Imminent: likely to happen soon

Overwrought: anxious, agitated

Relentless: never stopping

Torrential: violent, rapid, like a torrent

Transgression: sin, crime, wrongdoing

Some questions to ask yourself:

? How would you feel if you had tried hard to carry out a task you found difficult, but then someone came and told you that you were no good at doing that job?

? What does your school or your family do for others in need? Do you do your bit to help too?

? How does it feel to be generous or useful to others who need help?

? Do you ever catch yourself gossiping unkindly about other people?

? Do you ever repeat gossip about other people? Why do you think some people do this?

? Do you like it when other people gossip about you? If not, why not?

STORY 22

Modesty and Simplicity

WHEN MOTHER MADE HER CHOICE

When my mother was a young woman of eighteen, she had still not found a suitable husband. Her family was quite concerned about this, because it was the custom for girls to be betrothed*, or even married, when they reached twelve or thirteen years of age. My mother was a beautiful young woman, so I am told. The reason she had not found a husband was not because she was unattractive, in fact many suitors* had come her way, but she did not like any of them.

She would stamp her foot and say, "No, Father, I will not take that young man for a husband. He may have plenty of money and good prospects, but I do not like him. He is too proud." Or, "He is too vain."

It was always these faults that my mother seemed to find in her suitors.

"Ah, he thinks he is so clever!" she would say and then turn her back and walk out.

"Him! He thinks he is so handsome. He is more interested in impressing me with his appearance than in getting to know me. No, Father, not him!"

Or, "Him! All he does is strut to and fro with his head held high, expecting others to run hither and thither for him. No, not him!" And so on.

Her father and mother were exasperated[*]. Then one day, my father came to visit the house. He was a good-looking young man, clever and sensitive. When he met my mother he smiled and dropped his eyes. She watched the way he carried out his meeting and discussion with her father. It was temple business and she herself was very interested in that sort of thing. When he departed again, he looked modestly at her and smiled, saying his goodbyes.

"Now that is a young man I could marry," announced my mother to her parents that evening.

They were dumbfounded[*]. When eventually her mother could speak, she said, "But he's almost like a priest! He wears no fashionable clothes. He came here on foot, not on horseback; he brought no servants with him. He talks rather quietly for a self-assured man. Don't you want someone with more to offer, someone who is more outgoing, more flamboyant*, someone who would be more entertaining to be with?"

"Mother," replied her daughter, "you have supplied me with a string of raucous*, fancy young men and I have rejected them all. They are too bound up with their own importance. I want a man who is modest and whose life is one of simplicity, then I will be able to express myself as his wife and not become just another of his possessions."

"Very well," said her father, "I shall make enquiries about the young man."

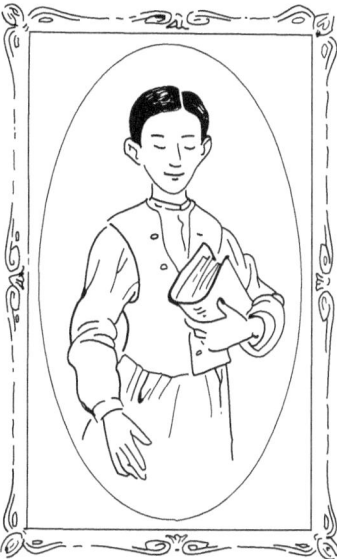

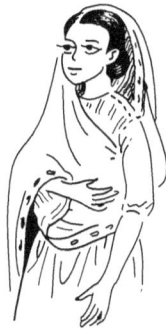

The two were married within six months. They were a perfect match. My mother's family never had cause to regret the union. After all, I was one of the products of it, was I not?

⊕

Some questions to ask yourself about modesty and simplicity:

? What do you feel about people who brag about their abilities, achievements or possessions?

? If you find yourself boasting, how do you feel about yourself, and how do your friends take it?

? How important is being beautiful or handsome compared to being a good, caring and honest friend?

STORY 23

Prayer and Meditation

THE OLD SCRIBE AND HIS TATTERED PARCHMENT

When my father, Rajendra, was a young man, his life was rather different from mine. He was born into a large family and, although they were *Brahmins**, they were not well off. They were the poor relations. However, Father was a clever man and he worked his way up to a good position in the temple. He was in charge of the ancient writings and he would have to copy them out when required by the priests and local dignitaries*.

He developed a beautiful style of writing. He would use the very best parchment*, which he obtained from a craftsman some distance away. He would always get edgy when his supplies began to run low and he would endeavour* to discover who would be going to the town where the parchment maker lived. He would ask them either

134

to be a carrier, or simply to get a message to the man that he needed his supplies to be replenished*.

On one occasion, the Great Festival of *Shakti* was approaching and he always needed to supply a number of people with written prayers for this event. His parchment was running low and nobody seemed to want to go to the town of the craftsman. Father became desperate. He asked the other scribes whether they had any spare parchment and one of them suggested asking old Ramchand, because he was ill and certainly would not be doing any scribing for a while yet. Father winced*. He knew that old Ramchand was quite capable of using the skin of an old goat to write upon. However he did not seem to have much choice. Ramchand's parchment it would have to be, as nobody else was willing to part with any. Old Ramchand smiled his toothless smile as he handed over a dog-eared* pile of sheets.

"Well, well, son," the old man said. "It's not quite up to your usual standard, is it? But do not forget that it is not the quality of paper that matters when people are praying, but the quality of the prayer itself. If we pray with an open heart, welcoming God into our lives, then that is all that is required. It is the same with meditation. You sit and you close your eyes and to all the

135

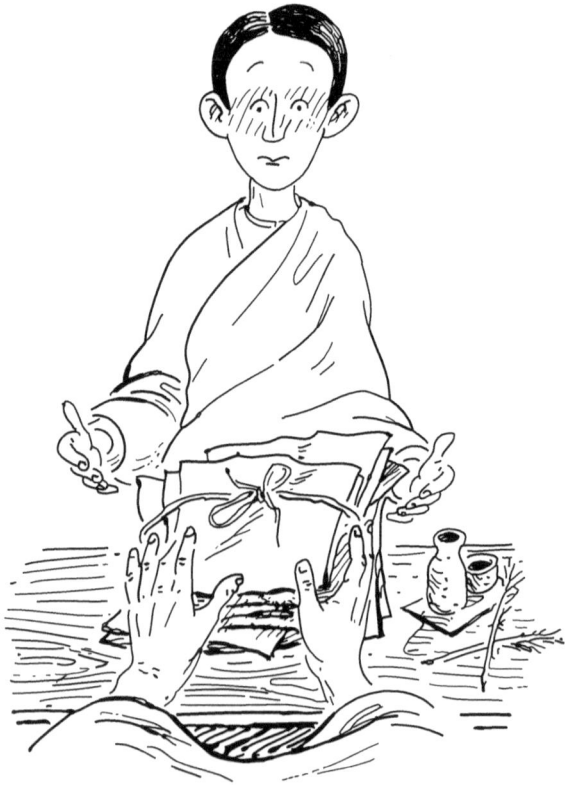

world you look as if you are meditating, but your mind may be filled with all manner of things. You may be thinking about your lovely wife to be, or that horse you are trying to purchase. You may be wondering what is to be served at the next meal. Nobody knows but you and God. It is always the quality of the prayer or the meditation that counts and not how it is presented. Wouldn't you agree, Rajendra?"

With that, my father humbly accepted the kind old scribe's sheets and set about making a special effort to get the words beautifully written, hoping that the devotees* would not notice the paper, and knowing that if they did it would not matter anyway.

$\oplus$

NEW WORDS:

Brahmins: members of the upper class in India, often priests

Devotees: serious followers of the services in the temple

Dignitaries: those who hold a high office or rank

Dog-eared: page corners of a book folded back like dogs' ears

Endeavour: to try hard, to make an earnest effort

Parchment: a material like paper made from the skins of sheep and goats

Replenished: refilled, restocked

Winced: shrank suddenly back or away

Some questions to ask yourself on prayer and meditation:

? When you need help, have you tried finding a quiet place and simply describing the problem and asking God for help?

? Have you ever tried sitting or lying down quietly and filling your mind with a beautiful picture, for example of a rose, or a moonlit lake, for five minutes? That would be a simple meditation, which would be calming and uplifting.

A story to illustrate unselfish action, self-sacrifice and giving help to others

FATHER SAVES A DROWNING WOMAN

I remember the occasion so well; it could have been yesterday. We were out on a family picnic down by the holy river. This was something that my family liked to do in the dry season, when we would be feeling very hot and dusty. We would take food and mats and, in the cooler part of the day, we would set ourselves up on the riverbank and watch the comings and goings. The children would bathe. Mother never would, but she would always paddle. Father taught us how to swim because, as he said, "If you fall into water, you will drown if you do not swim!"

My mother announced that she did not plan to fall into water. In fact she had decided that she would never fall into water!

"Sometimes there is no choice, my dear," said Father.

His words turned out to be prophetic*. Watching the boats running up and down the river, some rafts, some canoes and other larger rowing boats, we noticed a group of people suddenly stand up in their boat. It was quite near the shore, so we could see the expressions on their faces. They looked horror-struck. The women started to scream and the men to shout. There must have been half a dozen of them. The boat tipped at an angle and began to sink. The passengers all fell into the water and most started to swim around. Two of them managed to turn the boat upside down to hang on to; meanwhile three of them started swimming towards the shore.

It was very confusing. My father spotted something he did not like the look of. Quick as a flash he tore off his shoes and his jacket. He waded into the water and swam, faster than I have ever seen him swim, towards the boat, which was upstream from us.

"Daddy, Daddy!" we all screamed, not understanding what was going on. As he neared the boat, he reached out and pulled what looked like a rag from the water; attached to it was a woman, half drowned. He held her in one arm,

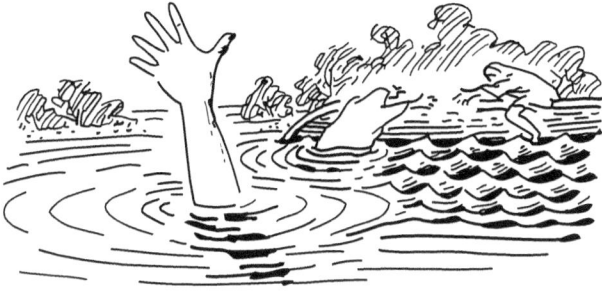

with her mouth above the surface of the water, and swam laboriously* back to the shore.

He dragged her out of the water and lay her on her front. She was promptly sick, then she started to breathe in huge, irregular gasps of air.

"It's all right. It's all right. You'll be fine now," Father was saying.

My mother held the woman tight in her arms and rocked her like she used to rock us when we were babies. Between them they both managed to calm the poor woman.

Finally the whole party was assembled on the bank. The woman had recovered her composure* enough to stand supported by her husband, who was thanking my father profusely*.

"If you had not been watching us and had not had the courage to swim out to us, my wife would have drowned!" he said. "I cannot thank you enough, sir!"

"Give your thanks to the Lord, my good man," said Father, embarrassed at all the attention. "It is He who decided that your wife should live today."

"Maybe, but if you had not been so unselfish, risking your own life, she would not have been saved!"

"Well, well," said Father. "Now you see children, why it is so important to learn to swim. You do it so you can save others from drowning!"

The party of wet day-trippers managed to raise a laugh and turned to make their way back to town. We packed up our picnic and walked back to the house, all holding on to a part of Father, so that he found it rather difficult to carry the basket.

Father looked down at us and said, "One day, maybe the Lord will ask you to risk your life for someone. You do have to think quite hard about it. In this case I knew I could swim out there and save the woman, but sometimes one has to allow others to die if certain death is going to be the outcome* for the rescuer."

NEW WORDS:

Composure: self-control, calmness

Laboriously: with difficulty

Outcome: result

Profusely: many times

Prophetic: foretelling future events

Self-sacrifice: giving up your personal
   interests for the benefit of others

Unselfish: thinking about others, not
   putting yourself first

Some questions to ask yourself about unselfish action and self-sacrifice:

? Think of the people who are close to you.
Think of some of the times when they have
given their time and attention willingly, instead
of doing what they wanted to do. How
important is that to you?

? Think of occasions when you have given your
time and energy unselfishly to other people.
How did it make you feel? How did they feel?

GLOSSARY

Abstinence: when a person chooses not to satisfy their appetites, e.g. for certain foods, drugs, alcohol or sexual activities

Academic: having to do with school or what you learn in school

Accumulate: to pile up, collect, gather

Adorning: decorating

Almighty (the): God

Antagonistic: against, not wanting to

Apologetically: wanting to say sorry

Arundada: Grandfather Arun

Austerity: being very stern or serious

Avidly: keenly

Betrothed: engaged to be married

Bewildered: confused or puzzled

Bounty: the wonderful gifts of nature

Brahma: the senior god; his job was creation

Brahmin: members of the upper class in India,

often priests

Caste: class, rank

Charitable: kind, considerate, generous

Chaste: 'pure', a virgin, innocent of sex

Cleanse: to remove dirt from, to remove guilt from

Community service: helping others where you live for no payment

Compassion/compassionate: kindness, kind-hearted, understanding

Composure: self-control, calmness

Condemned: to be called wrong

Condiments: the kinds of food that add flavour to a dish, e.g. salt, pepper, herbs, spices

Consequences: results

Constructive: valuable, practical, beneficial

Demurely: shyly, modestly

Denial: saying 'No', or refusing to enjoy the material pleasures of life, e.g. money, fashion, married life, extravagant food

Deprive: to take away from

Deputation: a group of people gathered to represent someone who is complaining

Devotees: serious followers of the services in the temple

Dharma: a person's correct path in life

Dignitaries: those who hold a high office or rank

Diminishes: makes smaller

Discomfiture: feeling worried, anxious or confused

Dismissive: sending away, not giving consideration to another person's comments

Distraught: anxious, worried, upset

Donned: put on

Dumbfounded: astonished, amazed

Earnest: serious, purposeful

Emanating: coming from

Encountered: met

Endeavour: to try hard, to make an earnest effort

Endure/endurance: withstand, bear up against, survive

Enveloped: wrapped, surrounded

Exasperated: greatly annoyed after losing patience with someone or something

Fetlock: the part just above a horse's hoof

Fisticuffs: fighting with fists

Flamboyant: exceptionally showy or dashing in one's speech, manner or appearance

Forbear/forbearance: to 'put up with' patiently

Harangue: to complain loudly

Illuminated: illustrated, having pictures

Imminent: likely to happen soon

Inclination: leaning towards, preference

Initially: at first

Inflated: puffed up (e.g. with pride)

Integrity: when someone is known to be honest they 'have integrity'

Intolerant: not being able to bear or to put up with other people's opinions and actions

Intoxicating: absolutely delightful, something which makes you feel drunk

Intrusive: nosey, inquisitive

Katha: The *Katha Upanishad* is a selection of Hindu verses in which freedom from desire is discussed

Laboriously: with difficulty, hard, strenuous

Latrines: toilets for use by many

Limited resources: only a certain amount of...

Lord Rama: perhaps the most virtuous hero in Hindu Mythology; a god in the Hindu religion

Magistrate: a judge

Meagre: poor, small, not enough

Namaste: a greeting of respect made to another person; the hands are held in the prayer position in front of the chest

Obedience: doing what you are told

Observing: watching with care

Outburst: a sudden explosion of strong feeling, such as anger

Outcome: result

Overarches: includes, encompasses

Overwrought: disturbed by worry, agitated

Paltry: small, worthless

Parchment: a material like paper made from the skins of sheep and goats

Penance: a penalty, something you do to make up for wrongdoing

Permeate: spread through

Perpetrator: a person who does something wrong

Profusely: many times

Prophetic: foretelling future events

Pursuits: activities

Quizzically: puzzled, expressing doubt, confusion or questioning

Railed: complained bitterly

Reconcile: to adjust

Regulate: to control by rules

Remarked: commented, said

Renunciation: giving up or rejecting something, e.g. worldly pleasures, family life

Replenished: refilled, restocked

Resentment: displeasure, bitterness, anger

Resolve: firm decision

Restriction: something that limits or restricts

Retribution: punishment that happens as a result of wrongdoing

Reverie: daydream

Sadhu: a Hindu monk

Sanyasin: a Hindu holy man

Scriptures: holy books

Self-gratification: pleasing the senses, satisfying your own desires

Self-sacrifice: giving up your personal interests for the benefit of others, or from a sense of duty

Shakti: Hindu goddess

Shamefacedly: expressing shame, embarrassed

Shiva: the great Hindu god of building up and destruction

Sincerely, sincerity: (with) genuine honesty

Slaughtered: killed

Soporific: causing sleep or drowsiness

Squabble: argue over small things

Stiffen your sinews: become strong

Struck dumb: without a voice

Substantial: solid, concrete or serious

Suitor: a man seeking to marry a woman

Summoned: asked to come

Taboo: forbidden

Take stock of: to consider, assess

Tolerance: being 'willing to accept' other people's ideas and questions

Torrential: violent, rapid, like a torrent

Tranquillity: calmness, peacefulness, serenity

Transformation: a major change

Transgression: sin, crime, wrongdoing

Transpired: came to light, became known

Unsavoury: unpleasant, distasteful

Unselfish: thinking about others, not putting yourself first

Unstable: unsettled, unpredictable

Unsuspecting: trusting

Unsympathetic: not being understanding and kind

Upanishads: a collection of very old religious texts from India

Victor: winner

Wan: weak and ill looking

Wince/winced: to shrink suddenly back or away

Wistful: a vague longing

Wryly: humorously (twisted or dry humour)

⊕

ABOUT THE WRITER
AND
THE BOOK

This book came to me as an answer to a prayer.

I was out of my depth in my yoga teaching. I knew there was more to learn, and that after fifteen years of teaching yoga I felt I was not progressing and neither were my students. I wanted to teach them about the '*Chakras*', the energy centres invisible to most people, that affect our daily lives, but I had no idea how to set about it. In those days there was nothing online, and very little information in books.

As I sat in meditation asking for help in preparing my next yoga lesson, an Indian *guru* came into my mind. This same *guru* had appeared to me once before when I was asking a question on spiritual matters. I was open to the idea of help arriving.

He said: "There is no point in teaching people about spiritual matters unless they are following the *Yamas* and *Niyamas* [the rules of life]."

I could not remember what all of the rules were, though I had learnt them many years previously when studying on my British Wheel of Yoga Teachers' training course.

The *guru* sternly told me off! "You should know the *Yamas* and *Niyamas*, you are a Yoga Teacher!" he said severely. Then he changed his manner and became kind and patient. "Never mind, don't worry, I'll help you," he said.

On that day, in the Launceston Leisure Centre in the UK, one hour before my next yoga class, much to my surprise and amazement, the *guru* gave me a little story about greed. It was about his own life when, as a small child, he learnt about sharing food from his father.

I was about forty-five at the time and hadn't written any stories since I'd been at school. I had followed a scientific route and become a biology teacher. Nothing was further from my mind than writing stories.

The following day, I asked for another story, on another of the rules of life: non-violence. It was like the first story: quirky, light-hearted, but making a point. I found that each time I asked for a story one came onto the paper. It was like mental dictation. I never knew what was going to be said next; no planning or thought was involved at all. I just needed to be fresh and alert and in a receptive state of meditation.

I soon gathered the first ten stories, which were about the main *Yamas* and *Niyamas*. I used them to help me teach my classes. They were a useful aid for me, as many of my yoga class members were older and wiser than I was, and I felt it would be embarrassing for me to try to tell them how to behave. The stories did it for me.

I was charmed by the guru's stories. The name Ramesh Guptananda formed in my mind when I asked what he was called. I discovered from my yoga reading that there was another set of ten more *Yamas* and *Niyamas*. Intrigued, I asked for stories on those subjects and they came.

Then life got in the way of story writing. I had a smallholding and six yoga and fitness classes and a family to attend to. However, one winter I decided to put the stories into context by considering the 'Eight Limbs of Yoga', of which, as we climb up the yogic tree to enlightenment, the *Yamas* and *Niyamas* are on the first branch, or limb.

I collected the Eight Limbs stories and then went on to ask Guptananda for stories to illustrate the *Chakras*. Finally, I asked for stories on the three *Gunas*, or states of being. Those were my last stories on yoga subjects. (They will be in my next book.) I created an online book containing all forty-three stories in 2008. This year, 2019, I am editing that book and splitting it into two. Technology has moved on and my online book is no longer working perfectly.

After writing the Guptananda stories, I found that if I meditated and asked for a story on a specific subject, I would be given one from anywhere in the world. I did not choose where the story should come from, but the guides came forward to tell me their stories. They came from far and wide: from China, Australia, Russia, America, Africa, India, France, Alaska to name just a few.

I created an educational story blog, yogastories. wordpress.com in order to offer my stories to the world, and indeed they are used by people from many English-speaking nations, and by teachers from all over the world who need simple stories in English to help their students learn the language.

If you have enjoyed *The Great Little Book of Yoga Stories: Book One*, spread the word and look out for Book Two and perhaps more books on therapeutic and social or values education, to be published after Book One.

AFTERWORD

Swami Shivapremananda

Swami Shivapremananda is an Indian-born man who was the foremost *Swami*, or teacher, of the British Wheel of Yoga for many years.

Facts and fiction are a part of life. Within it, as this manuscript illustrates, a basic spiritual philosophy is interwoven to emphasise the real goal of yoga. The orientation being Indian, the mythical figure transforms himself in these pages as *Swami* Ramesh Guptananda. It is the responsibility of the reader to sift the reality from fiction, and imbibe the true spirit of the book.

Profound philosophical teachings are expressed through stories, which is a good way to relate to the reader. Even though this work is written with the younger generation in view, it has a general appeal overall. The text is based on Patanjali's *Yogasutras*, also comprehensively called *Ashtanga* yoga.

Tessa Hillman's personal life-stories are interestingly illustrative. The foundation of all the branches of yoga is *Yama* and *Niyama*, or the ten ethical and regulatory disciplines. They should play a vital role among all those who practise and teach yoga.

The truth of a theory is in its viability through application, and the purpose of an ideal is to make an idea real. Without pragmatism, an ideal remains sterile.

The four main branches of yoga are *Gyana*, *Bhakti*, *Raja* and *Karma*. They are essentially synthetic in their practice, although one can be more predominant as per the individual's predisposition.

Dhyana yoga is an adjunct to *Raja* yoga, as is *Hatha* yoga.

However Patanjali does not mention *asana* and *pranayama* as a system of physical culture, but as fixed sitting postures and regulated breathing, preparatory to meditation. By itself, *Hatha* yoga does not help in spiritual progress. In spite of their popularity worldwide, the practice of *asana* and *pranayama* alone does not make one a yogi. It is ridiculous that in the West some yoga students and

160

teachers just do that, revealing their limited knowledge of yoga.

Being a yogi means a lot. It is a life-long process of integration of the body, mind and soul, as the term yoga implies.

I have known Tessa for quite a few years; reading this draft, which she sent me for writing the Foreword, I find that she has done a good job.

Buenos Aires, Argentina
21 June 2002

⊕

Swami Shivapremananda is a real live *guru*, who helped, encouraged, lectured and taught hundreds of yoga students in Britain and abroad. Indian born, in 1925, in West Bengal, to a family of the *Brahmin* caste, he was educated at a Jesuit school as a boy. He graduated from Calcutta University with a degree in politics and history, then he entered the ashram of the Divine Life Society at Rishikesh, where he studied and taught for sixteen years. He had no time for self-styled *swamis* and told me a *swami* is a spiritual teacher who has studied under a *guru* at an *ashram* for at least twelve years.

He emigrated initially to the US and ran many

yoga classes in various places. He established three *ashrams* in South America and spent his last thirty years living and teaching in those places in Santiago, Chile; Buenos Aires, Argentina and Montevideo, Uruguay. He placed much emphasis in his work on *Karma* yoga, service to the poor, and of course to his students. He was the foremost *swami*, or teacher, of the British Wheel of Yoga for many years. The BWY is the largest regulatory body in the UK, which governs the training of yoga teachers and promotes the purposes and values of yoga.

I was privileged to have *Swami* Shivapremananda to stay at my house for a week on two separate occasions, while he was on his regular annual teaching tours in the UK. I asked him if he would mind reviewing my book. I was unsure whether he would consider it to be of any merit, however he graciously agreed. He did not share my beliefs about spirit guides, it seems, not having had any personal experience of such entities, however he did like the book. A writer of many books on yoga himself, he was a modest, quiet, rigorous man, highly self-disciplined, and a great inspiration to so many of us students and teachers of yoga. I am most grateful to him for taking the trouble to read my book and write an Afterword for me.

I will not attempt to define the yogic terms in this

Afterword, that is for the student and practitioner of yoga to do. Some of the terms refer to the material in Book Two, to be published in 2020.

ACKNOWLEDGEMENTS

First of all, I would like to thank my husband of thirty-one years, Gerry Hillman, for his support, tolerance and patience over the seven years it took to create this book. We are now no longer together, but are still supportive of what we each do. After I wrote the first draft of the book there were long periods of not writing, when I felt I needed to be earning money. There were times when I wondered how I would ever be able to finish the work, but convinced of its importance, I pressed on when I could. My Aunt Jean Fife actually made it possible for me to finish the book, by being a very frugal lady. She left some money to my mother who, similarly frugal, left it to my brothers and to me. So I send my grateful thanks to them both, although they are in spirit now.

Many thanks also to Philip Jewell; dear yoga friend and advisor, willing to share my trials and tribulations, giving me his quiet counsel whenever I asked for it. Philip edited my book in the early days and again when the new material had been added.

I have also received help and encouragement from my editors Brian Davis, Carole Alderman, Jean Reynolds, Rosie Barratt and Renu Gidoomal, all of whom looked carefully through the book and suggested adjustments according to their own expertise and background.

Dr Shastry, the late Academic Director of the Bhavan Institute of Indian Culture in London, taught *Sanskrit* and Hindu Philosophy. He checked the book both for accuracy with regard to the Indian way of life, and for its interpretation of Hindu Philosophy and *Sanskrit*.

Helen Greathead edited the second edition published in 2019. Maggie Robshaw helped with the proof reading.

I would also like to thank Patrick Gamble, a psychic artist. I had never met him, though his work was recommended to me, and having seen his lovely pictures, I asked him for a picture of my spirit guide. Patrick, knowing nothing at all about me, saw Guptananda as clear as day and painted a beautiful portrait of him. Patrick, being psychic, also told me that I had been working with the *guru* on spiritual matters and that many sheets of paper were involved! I was able to tell Patrick that he was correct!

I would also like to include in my thanks my husband, Dr David Guiterman, whom I married in 2014, a scientist to the core, who is quietly intrigued by what I am writing. His reaction: "They are delightful stories, innocent and simple, and seem very Indian. The language in them does not sound at all like you."

That provoked a 'whew' from me!!

B.K.S. Iyengar, through his book *Light on Yoga,* has been a very important source of information for me throughout my years as a yoga teacher. I would like to express my appreciation of his work.

My dear friend the late Alan Nisbet deserves many thanks. His wonderful illustrations enliven the book and I love them! Sally Atkins drew beautifully the undisciplined horses of Story 12.

This book would not have been published if it were not for the help of the above people, but it would never have happened at all had not *Swami* Ramesh Guptananda come into my mind and given me the stories, for which I am eternally grateful.

Thanks to Bek Pickard for text layout, and Mick Clough (handmade-media.co.uk) for cover design.

Top of the Village Publishing

https://topofthevillagepublishing.co.uk

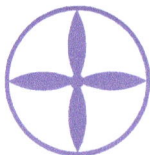

www.ingramcontent.com/pod-product-compliance
Lightning Source LLC
Chambersburg PA
CBHW041214030426
42336CB00023B/3346